"Rarely does one find such a storehouse of useful information compiled into one handy resource. This guide to establishing a terrific practice is destined to become your go-to reference for those interested in improving the patient experience."

—Paul Klotman, MD, President & CEO, Baylor College of Medicine

"Michael Harris has written a primer for doctors who want to survive financially in a competitive and ever-changing market. His knowledge and wisdom have been gained through years of personal experience in both a successful private practice and as an institutional leader. The writing is clear, practical, and uniquely fills the gaps in expertise of many physicians."

—Lawrence Smith, MD, Dean, Hofstra North Shore-LIJ School of Medicine

"Physicians spend years training to be the very best at delivering excellent medical care to our patients. Unfortunately, most of us spend little more than several hours, if that, learning all that we need to learn to keep our practices alive and thriving. In this age of rapidly changing medical delivery and reimbursement systems, physicians must make it our duty to be well informed about the business of practicing medicine. Michael Harris's new book, *Excellence with an Edge: Practicing Medicine in a Competitive Environment*, is an excellent compilation of practical information and astute business strategies for building and growing your practice. This book is a must-read for every physician and office manager. We owe it to our patients and ourselves to learn this information if we plan to continue to provide care for our patients. I know my partners will each be getting a copy of this book to be read before our next practice meeting."

—James D. Capozzi, MD, Chairman, Department of Orthopaedic Surgery, Winthrop University Hospital

"Great medical care and great practice management require two entirely different skill sets. Yet you can't provide the former without the latter—not for long, anyway. Dr. Harris has written a book that teaches physicians how to grow a strong, vibrant, financially sound practice. Best of all, he explains it in a way that inspires rather than overwhelms. His easy-to-grasp directives empower us to fulfill our purpose—healing our patients—while still paying our bills and, yes, ourselves."

—Robert E. Kelly, MD, Group Senior Vice President, Chief Medical Officer and Chief Operating Officer, NewYork-Presbyterian/Columbia

Excellence with an Edge is a must-read for any physician in leadership or striving to be in a leadership position. Dr. Harris brilliantly combines the financial acumen that is required to run a successful practice with the service principles that create loyal patients and referring physicians."

—Matt Kalaycio, MD, FACP, Co-Director, Bone Marrow Transplant Program; Director, Chronic Leukemia and Myeloma Program, Cleveland Clinic Taussig Cancer Institute, Cleveland, Ohio; Professor, Department of Medicine, Cleveland Clinic Lerner College of Medicine of Case Western Reserve University, Cleveland, Ohio

"Dr. Harris has written a lively and creative book. He shares his personal experience to give insight into managing a successful medical practice. This book is practical, sensible, and appealing to clinicians in a wide range of practices."

—Stephen Dolgin, MD, Chief Pediatric Surgery, Cohen Children's Medical Center of New York; Professor of Surgery and Pediatrics, Hofstra NS-LIJ School of Medicine

EXCELLENCE
WITH AN
edge

PRACTICING MEDICINE IN A
COMPETITIVE ENVIRONMENT

MICHAEL T. HARRIS, MD

Published by:
Fire Starter Publishing
913 Gulf Breeze Parkway, Suite 6
Gulf Breeze, FL 32561
Phone: 850-934-1099
Fax: 850-934-1384
www.firestarterpublishing.com

ISBN: 978-0-9840794-9-0

Library of Congress Control Number: 2010936296

Printed in the United States of America

To Debbie, Rebecca, and Sam, whose love, support, and sacrifice give me my edge.

TABLE OF CONTENTS

· · · · · · · · · ·

FOREWORD

· · · · · · · · · ·

This is a challenging time for physicians. As the landscape of healthcare changes, it has never been more important for physicians to know the business side of medicine. Getting this right will give you the edge needed to create the best patient experience, and isn't that why you got into this in the first place?

Consider the following true stories. They show just how important the business side of a medical practice really is.

Story #1: I was working in a hospital when I started to notice that a certain doctor came around each day a little before noon. It seemed like one hospital leader or another would always go to lunch with him, and his lunch was always charged to administration. Later I found out why. His practice was so far behind in billing and collecting that he had major cash flow issues—so many that he needed to have his meal paid for every day.

It reminds me of a picture I saw that showed a physician on the side of the road holding a sign that read, "Will operate for food."

Story #2: A multi-specialty group practice of 28 physicians moved out of their space and built a very nice facility. They also each signed an agreement to cover the debt. Before long, things began to get rough. To their surprise, some of the physicians found out that even if they left the practice, they were still liable for the debt. In less than two years, they had gone from holding an exciting open house to selling the facility and their practice and becoming employees of a hospital in exchange for a portion of accounts receivable and assumption of some debt.

I am not suggesting that being employed by the hospital is in any way undesirable. What is unfortunate is that these physicians allowed poor decisions and weak operations to create a situation in which the group had no leverage.

Story #3: A young physician signed an agreement to work for a health-care organization. The first year's salary was guaranteed, and the organization was to run the administrative function so the physician could focus on patient care. Life could not have been better. That is, it couldn't have been better until the end of year one when the salary became a draw, and a disagreement took place regarding collections, expenses, productivity, and so forth.

Here's the point of all three stories: No matter what type of practice a physician works in, it is vital that he or she knows what a well-run practice looks and feels like.

Once you know how the numbers work (and they are working for you), the focus becomes the patient again. Dr. Harris lays the foundation to help you build a competitive edge that will create loyalty in patients and physicians alike. *Excellence with an Edge* takes you full circle to focusing on caring for the patient.

At the end you'll even get a glimpse of what excellence looks like from the eyes of the referring physicians, office staff, and patients.

If you are a practice manager, you will want every physician you work with to study this book. It will make the practice run better.

If you are a vendor to a practice, you also will want to make sure every physician reads this book. Your life will be better.

And, of course, if you are a physician, you will want to read this book. Think of it as your treatment plan for a healthy practice.

Studer Group's mission is to create better organizations for patients to receive care, for staff to work, and for physicians to practice medicine. Excellence with an Edge achieves each of those goals.

Whoever first made the statement, "What you don't know won't hurt you," obviously never practiced medicine. What you don't know will not only hurt you, the physician, but it will also hurt your family, your patients, your colleagues, and everyone whose life intersects with yours.

I hope you will read and learn from Dr. Harris's excellent book. It will help you operate a more successful practice—and enjoy more control over your work and life.

Quint Studer
Founder & CEO, Studer Group

INTRODUCTION

· · · · · · · · · ·

My Edge

One of my earliest childhood memories is that of my brother's pinky jammed into my cheek as he said, "Wanna bet? Wanna bet? Wanna put some money on that?"

I rarely did want to bet with him, and on those occasions when I did, I almost always lost. Of course, he was destined to go on to a highly successful career on Wall Street, so he obviously had a knack for money and betting. In fact, when we were teenagers, my brother would often talk about business and finance with our father at the dinner table. I tuned it all out because I was going to be a doctor. And by then I was much bigger than my brother, so he no longer dared touch me.

I believed that all I needed to know was that I was going to take care of patients and make their lives better. I was a "people person." And accordingly, I felt that I was not going to "debase" myself by discussing or learning about money. I only wish that my father had smacked me on the forehead back then and said, "You moron! You need to know this stuff. Everybody needs to know this stuff! And get a haircut!"

When I got married during the fourth year of medical school, my financial knowledge had not advanced a whit. My wife and I moved into an apartment that we just kind of lucked into...which felt a lot like how my career in surgery began.

About a year before I completed my surgical residency, while I was in the operating room one day, I got a message out of the blue that "the big guy" had called and would like me to call him at home. "The big guy" was one of the senior partners of *the* surgical practice in New York City, the one you secretly daydreamed about, but never really imagined joining. He was a giant, in so many ways. As a surgeon, he was gifted in terms of skill and the knowledge of his craft. His patients, colleagues, residents, and students worshiped him. He knew everybody in the hospital by name, including the people who cleaned the floors, and treated each person as if nothing else mattered at any given time. In short, he was the consummate physician.

My first thought was #$*! There's something wrong! I wondered if I had forgotten to dictate a case of his or if something bad had happened to one of his patients. When I did call him back that night, I nearly fell off my chair. He said, "We want to take you out for dinner and talk to you about what you're going to be doing after next year and for the rest of your life."

Dinner was a whirlwind. The partners painted a picture of a dream practice that I was being tapped to join. Up until that point, my plan had been to hang out a shingle in the suburbs and be a gentleman surgeon in a nice, private practice...not that I had any idea how to go about such a thing.

The conversation that night was focused on all kinds of things...like the philosophy of their practice...what my future would look like as a part of their group...and how I was the right man to help carry the group's rich tradition forward. I was blown away. The subject of money came up only once, almost as an aside. There would be plenty of money, they said.

I never saw a lawyer, and although there was a contract, I was a full partner long before any of us ever signed it. That wouldn't quite work today, and I would definitely not recommend such a course.

The instructions my new partners gave me on how to succeed in my medical practice were very few and really quite basic. One told me, "The only thing you have to remember is the three A's: Be Affable, Able, and Available. Of the three, make sure you're available."

Another partner instructed me to take excellent care of the referring doctors, in addition to the patients. He urged me to make their concerns mine, to ensure their satisfaction and continued referrals. Essentially, he instructed me to allow a referring physician to feel that his burden had been lifted as soon as he completed his phone call with me. The referrer, he said, should be secure in the knowledge that I had assumed full responsibility for the patient's care—not just surgical care, but also non-surgical tests, family issues, and whatever else might come up. This was probably the most useful advice of all. (Today, we might call such advice "Acting like an owner, rather than a renter." I will re-visit this concept a number of times in the pages to come.)

One other piece of advice was a little more ominous. I was warned, "It takes months or years of great clinical outcomes to establish a good reputation... and just one mistake to establish a bad name." (Interesting advice, and while fortunately—thus far—not relevant to my own situation, I will review some key related issues in Chapter 7—"How to Destroy a Practice in 90 Days.")

Just before I started, I was introduced to the staff. We had an "office manager" in the practice—essentially a bookkeeper who had been promoted over the course of 20 years to her current position. An additional three full-time staff worked in the front of the office. Two full-time billing people, a medical assistant, and a night housekeeper rounded out the group.

I had no idea how these people came to be in the jobs that they were doing or, indeed, what it was they were supposed to be doing at all. This kind of information, as well as discussions about money, finance, and insurance, was never really part of my education when I joined the practice. Don't get me wrong. This was fine with me. I had no reason to care about these things. I was a doctor. I was the rookie in the busiest single surgical practice in New York City. I had grasped the brass ring, and nothing could have been better. I was getting paid what I thought was a reasonable amount of money, and the prospects of good times ahead were excellent.

So, when the year-end closing occurred in the last week of December that first year, I went with the flow. After two days of preparation, with papers flying all over the office, the group sat down to "settle up," with the office manager close at hand to track down any necessary documents. I was told really nothing, other than to bring my checkbook.

We all sat in the conference room, me with my checkbook, the other guys shuffling stacks of receipts and other documents. The managing partner had a legal pad with markings that only he could decipher. After five hours of reviewing the hard copy of all that had transpired over the previous year, they arrived at "the numbers."

I was told to write about nine different checks to five different people. In exchange, I received something like six different checks from three different people. I think that the checks I received amounted to more than the checks that I wrote, but I'm not absolutely certain of that. Finally, we all went out for a great dinner and drinks to celebrate our readiness for the next year to begin.

I survived three of those yearly closings. They required a great deal of time and effort, but in the end were fair, legal, and blessed by the accountant. The third one was my favorite, because after the exchange was over, I received checks that were demonstrably larger than the checks I wrote. I was a partner.

It was a great time in my life. I had two young babies, a burgeoning young practice, and a new life in the suburbs. While we had no real idea how to buy a house and evaluate a mortgage, my wife and I took the plunge anyway and went to contract on a new home, which was to close in early July.

But on June 30, exactly three years to the day that I had joined the practice, my mentor, "the big guy"—the giant, the rainmaker, and the managing partner—died. I could not have been more devastated. Besides my love for this man both personally and as a physician role model, I was days away from closing on a house that I suddenly was worried about not being able to afford.

In retrospect, his death was a major turning point early in my career. I was the junior man in a surgical practice that needed a new managing partner. That was when I realized that while patient care is and always will be paramount, part of being a doctor—a great doctor like my mentor—is owning and operating a business that allows us to do the things that we are trained to do. It was also the moment that I realized I had no idea what that entailed. Even worse, it occurred to me that I was practicing medicine on a small island (Manhattan) with more doctors than most countries have people, and that I was actually going to have to compete with them to succeed. Nobody ever told me that.

If you are reading this, you are already many steps ahead of where I was.

Fifteen years later, I am the vice chairman of surgery at a major academic medical center, with the responsibility of managing a 46-surgeon practice. I have one of the largest individual Inflammatory Bowel Disease (IBD) surgical practices in the country. I continue to make an excellent living. And, most importantly, I am consistently ranked in the 99th percentile nationally in overall patient satisfaction. I am also fortunate to be the recipient of Studer Group's 2009 Leadership in Medicine Award.

Here is my biggest secret: There are probably 20 surgeons within a 15-mile radius who could do what I do, just about as well as I do it. But you wouldn't necessarily know it by talking to patients, doctors, or even insurance companies, who continue to see me as *the* go-to surgeon for IBD. Please don't tell anybody.

What I have learned since the days of my mentor's death about building highly successful medical practices in an era of fierce competition is the subject of this book.

CHAPTER 1

FINDING YOUR EDGE
· · · · · · · · · · ·

Their Edge

I keep hearing about the current and impending physician shortage. I don't know about you, but I don't feel it. As I mentioned, I practice in New York City, which is a big, tough town. Places like New York, Chicago, L.A., Miami, and a thousand other big cities and towns are like seas teeming with wildlife… There are guppies, and there are whales, and everything in between. You think you're alone? You think you have a niche that no one else can service? You think you have a unique skill? Are you a guppy…or a whale?

Check out HealthGrades.com. If you're a gastroenterologist in Chicago, there are 370 others just like you within a 25-mile radius. Phoenix has 315 orthopedists. There are 304 cardiologists in Pittsburgh, and 634 ENT guys in New York.[1] Six hundred thirty-four! Okay, so there are no dermatologists in Wasilla, Alaska, but there are 66 hematologists in Indianapolis. Thirty-one colorectal surgeons in Cleveland. One hundred twenty-one family practice doctors in Wheeling, West Virginia. You want to relax? Go for the simple life? The retired life in Boca Raton, Florida? Well, if you're a urologist, there are 244 others willing and able to do your work. That's pretty sobering, isn't it?

And what is their edge? What is their competitive advantage over doctors like you and me? Well, besides sheer numbers and market saturation, there are a number of forces of which you need to be aware.

The first is consolidation. The era of the independent, solo practitioner, I believe, is just about over. Most independent practitioners have at least created single specialty groups, which, in and of themselves, have a hard time competing these days. The competition comes from huge, multi-specialty groups and/or faculty practices. Even many multi-specialty groups have given up their independence and become hospital-based or hospital-owned.

On a larger scale, individual hospitals have consolidated to create networks and huge health systems. In fact, hospitals and independent practitioners are closing their doors with increasing regularity in large markets like New York, Philadelphia, Boston, San Francisco, L.A., Chicago, and Miami. You get the picture.

It's easy to see where some of the competitive advantage comes from in this consolidated market. These large groups have much better access than you and I to funding for equipment, expansion, and other things that foster business. And the old saying is certainly true, "It takes money to make money." And, while perhaps from time to time you've had patients willing to donate a few thousand dollars here and there for your research projects or other professional endeavors, when was the last time you were able to secure a $10-million gift for your small private practice?

Large groups and systems have access to technologies that you cannot possibly afford. Yes, you can send your patients to use the machines and get the tests that these other entities own, but each time you do this, you are creating business for your potential competitors.

Large groups also have the ability to retain professional and non-professional support staff with expertise in business and management (the so-called "suits" that we, as a profession, used to hold in contempt). Consolidation also has led to the ability to aggressively market and create brand recognition for large multi-specialty groups and health systems. We'll discuss your ability to use marketing and brand recognition to your advantage in Chapter 5.

Before you dismiss this as lowbrow, it's worth looking at the results of a study from McKinsey & Company in 2007[2], in which they surveyed over 2,000 U.S. patients with commercial insurance or government plans. When asked if they have ever requested a specific hospital from their physician, an incredible 42 percent answered that they made specific requests from their doctor as to what hospital they wanted to be affiliated with. Another 28 percent discussed the choice of hospital with their doctor. See Figure 1.1 for that breakdown.

Figure 1.1: Patient Preferences for Hospitals

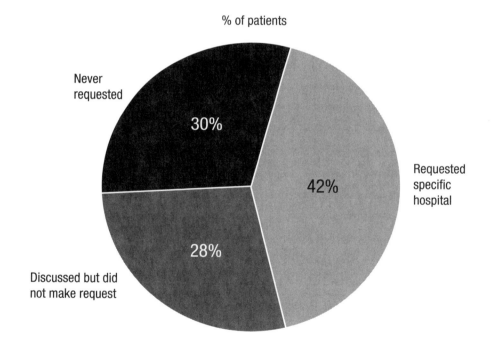

Have you ever requested a specific hospital from your physician?

% of patients

Never requested — 30%

Requested specific hospital — 42%

Discussed but did not make request — 28%

Source: McKinsey Quarterly, Nov. 2007

Another trend to be aware of is the growing number of accountable care organizations, or ACOs. ACOs are creating and sharpening their edge in order to take advantage of new payment models, some of which are buried in the new Patient Protection and Affordable Care Act (ObamaCare). These ACOs create a competitive model for the integration of care for certain diseases. They also stand to benefit from global reimbursements at higher rates than those of traditional organizations that bill for individual goods and services. Efficiency in these systems will create the potential for higher profit margins and a competitive advantage in securing patients.

ACOs, along with other large, integrated practices and health systems, are making use of expensive and complex electronic medical record systems to quickly disseminate best practices, which deliver efficient care and great outcomes. As a result, they have caught the eye of both commercial and government payers. One group, the Geisinger Health System, has gone so far as to guarantee outcomes. For example, if you are readmitted to one of the Geisinger hospitals within 90 days of a CABG, Geisinger will eat the cost. Are you ready to compete with that?

In addition to quality initiatives and marketing, systems like Geisinger (indeed every health system, including the hospital with which you are affiliated) are measuring patient perception of care with sophisticated surveys. In fact, they're measuring everything. As you will see later, this type of measurement and attention to patient and also physician satisfaction is critical to competing in this climate.

And finally, if the trend in early 2010 continues, weaker consumer demand for healthcare provides just one more reason that competition for patients will intensify. Just a year after insurers told us that healthcare usage was surging, utilization has dropped dramatically. The *Wall Street Journal*[3] attributes this to consumers forgoing elective procedures in a weak economy and fewer visits to primary care doctors and specialists as more unemployed lose their access to health insurance.

Figure 1.2: Patient Visits Decline

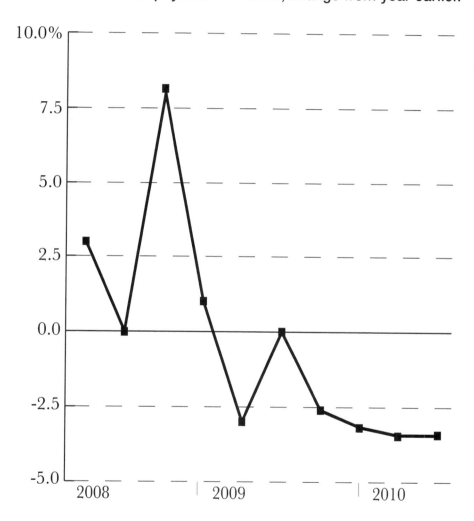

Patients' visits to physicians' offices, change from year earlier.

Source: UBS Investment Research analysis of IMS Health data

But do not despair. You can compete in this environment. You can not only survive, but thrive. I can help you be the whale in your waters rather than the guppy.

Your Edge

You are a specialist. Whether you are a neuro-ophthalmologist in Denver, Colorado, or a family practitioner in Grand Forks, North Dakota, you are a specialist in your field. The suggestion that primary care specialists somehow don't need to compete for business or share the same concerns as tertiary or quaternary care practitioners is a myth.

We all have expenses. We all have the need to bring in revenues that exceed those expenses by a margin great enough to allow us to make a living. We all feel the pressures of declining reimbursements and increased expenses and, of course, competition. We all have to get our patients from somewhere. So while the neurosurgeon may get most of his patients from the neurologist, and the neurologist may get most of her patients from the internist, the internist isn't just sitting in his office waiting for people to show up. He is a specialist, too, in every sense of the word, and must focus on his business in exactly the same ways.

It is worth remembering, as we reel from today's competitive reality, that the first thing patients choose is a doctor. While there is a trend towards consumerism, and patients do want to affiliate themselves with specific systems and hospitals and maybe even groups, at the end of the day what they really want is a great doctor. If you are that great doctor, and, as importantly, everybody knows it, then you have a tremendous edge.

Remember who you are and how you got here. I am willing to bet that compared to your ninth grade peers, you were smarter than most, more energetic than most, and more hardworking than most. Throughout your life as a child and young adult, you have succeeded in every single thing that you have done. You have risen above most, if not all, of your peers in school and in extracurricular pursuits (sports, music, art, whatever), and this success has propelled you in education to the highest levels in high school, college, and then graduate school. You didn't get where you are because you are lazy or stupid. Quite the opposite. Failure has never been an option, and there is no reason to believe that it is now.

In addition to all this, you care (or at least you once did) about the work that you do and the influence and impact that you have on other people's lives. If you have lost that spark, to any degree, it is time to get that passion back. And it applies not only to your patients but to the people in your workplace as well.

Whether you realize it or not, you are a leader, and you have the ability to use this to your advantage. You have what is known in politics as a sphere of influence over which you have the ability to exert control. Now, not everybody's sphere is as large as everybody else's. Clearly, if you are the CEO of a $5-billion health system, your influence extends to a larger group of people than if you are an employed physician just out of residency in a large faculty practice. And yet, if you are closer to the latter, as most of us are, please do not underestimate your ability to exert a great deal of influence over the people around you and to gain and maintain control of your environment.

It would be easy, particularly for the younger among us, or those of us who are small cogs in a large machine, to cede control to outside forces. I see this repeatedly in my own organization and others, and have likened it to a "victim mentality."

"Victim thinkers" tend to come up with one reason after another why they can't be successful—or why they won't reach this or that goal—and then they give up. Once you start practicing this deadly sin, it can be a very difficult habit to break. It renders you incapable of being successful.

Just recently, I had lunch with a friend of mine who is a renowned surgical sub-specialist. Over the years, he has been in practice in a variety of settings, including large faculty practices at several institutions, multi-specialty private practices, and single-specialty private practices. A couple of years ago, he returned to our faculty practice with much-deserved fanfare.

As we were having lunch, his cell phone rang, and he took a call directly from a patient. When he ended the call, he said, "Mickey, you're involved in administration, right? You've got to do something." (This is one of my favorite phrases: "You've got to do something!")

"I have to give everybody my cell phone number, because when patients call my office, nobody ever answers the phone. And when someone does answer the phone, they always tell people the wrong thing. I lose five cases a week because of the way the phones are answered. Five cases a week, and there are nine of us in the practice, so can you imagine? We're each losing five cases a week—that's forty-five cases a week that we're losing because of the phones. If we were able to capture those forty-five cases, the hospital, the medical school, and the entire faculty practice would never have financial problems again."

Somewhat amused, and skeptical, I asked him how long this had been going on. He said, "Two years." I asked him, "For two years, this has been going on? You have been losing all of these cases, every week, because of the way that people are answering or not answering your phones?" To which he said, "Right. Now can you fix this?"

I said, "Sure, I can try. Let me ask you a couple of questions. First, who answers your phones?"

He said, "What do you mean?"

And I said, "Who answers your phones? What is the name of the person or the names of the people who answer your phones? Are they your own people? Are they people in your division? Are they people from your department? Are they people from the medical school? Who are the people who answer your phones? That way I can help you resolve this."

This is when my friend, the world-renowned surgeon, lost his edge. "I think it's the department. That's it. The department has people who answer the phones."

I said, "Okay, good. Now, where do they do this? Where do they perform this function?" He asked, "What do you mean by that?"

And I said, "Well, do they sit in your office? Do they sit in a central location on your floor? Are they in this building? Are they on 74th Street? Are they in Texas or are they in a call center in India somewhere?"

All he could say was, "I don't know."

So I said, "My friend, you're really not going about this in the best way." (Let me tell you that what I actually said showed a great deal less tact and is probably unprintable.)

Then I said, "If something like this had happened to me once, just *once*, where a patient complained that he or she was unable to get through to my office, I would have done something about it. I wouldn't wait for five times a week for two years to then, in an off-the-cuff conversation with somebody else who's barely, peripherally related to my practice, have a conversation about it.

"If I were you, I would have, and I would now, first find out exactly who the people are who answer my phones, and find out where they are located. And I would go there, maybe even with a token gift in my hands: flowers, cookies, sandwiches, something. And I would introduce myself.

"I would say to the person or people who answer my phone, 'Hi. I'm Mickey Harris, one of the surgeons whose phones you answer. For the last 20 years, I have been helping to care for patients with Crohn's disease, ulcerative colitis, and other kinds of problems. Often, when my patients or their family members call the practice, they are anxious or worried or in great pain. So it's very important that the first voice they hear is a friendly and knowledgeable one, who assists them promptly. Your words and actions reflect greatly on me and what I do, so I really appreciate that you're helping me to care for them. Thank you for your efforts and your hard work.'"

Then I explained to my colleague that I also provide the people who handle my calls with written information, including scripts of the exact words that I want them to say when they answer the phones for my patients in a variety of different situations.

I encourage them to ask me any questions and to contact me at any time to further help them help me take care of our patients. And I would close our conversation by once again thanking them for the work that they do, connecting it again back to our original purpose, which is caring for people and their families. I told my friend that I guaranteed that if he would do this, that the nature and tenor of the phone answering for his practice would change immediately.

This is but one example of what I see all the time in a variety of different practice situations. Unfortunately, we as physicians have been taught the medicine, but not the customer service or management skills we need to succeed. Even through our residency training, we have been conditioned to care for the patients in a medical sense and to expect that everything else will be taken care of by somebody else, while in practice, nothing could be further from the truth.

Whether you have trained for it or not, whether you anticipated it or not (and I suspect you have not), you run a business. And yes, the primary product of your business is the care of patients, but this doesn't happen in a vacuum. I have found over the years that those of us in private practice get a sense of this the quickest. That doesn't mean that we're very good at operating our businesses, but at least we recognize that a great deal more goes into providing excellent care than showing up at the bedside or in the procedure room. Whether you are the CEO of a large group, a junior partner in a private practice, an employed physician in a huge multi-specialty group, or a hospital-based ER doc, you run a business.

You have staff who support you, whether you had a hand in hiring and training them or not. You spend money, utilize resources, and occupy valuable space, whether you are involved in the accounting for these resources or not. You have insurance. You follow policies and adhere to regulatory requirements, whether you pay attention to that or not.

Equally important, you perform work (the caring for patients) that can and must generate the revenues required to offset these expenses, with enough left over to cover the income you earn to provide for your family. And whether you participate in it or not, there's a whole lot of work that has to go on behind the scenes in order to transform the care you provide for Mrs. Smith into new shoes for your kids.

To succeed, and, yes, thrive, in today's competitive environment, you need to learn your business. Because of who you are—because of your background—you are much more capable of learning the business side of medical practice than the suits are at learning the medicine side. And when you do, you'll be that much more effective at exerting your influence over your environment, to both control and enlarge your sphere of influence and to maximize your income.

If any one of you reading this book does this, you will make your life and the lives of your patients, their families, and your family better. If all of you reading this book do this, you will not only make your lives better, but your spheres of influence will grow to such a degree that your institutions and the entire profession will gain.

You are clearly looking to take control. That is why you are reading this now. You have the intellect, the drive, and the ability to learn to use the tools to do this. This is your edge.

Finding Your Edge

As I noted earlier, my partner's sudden death on the last day of my third year in practice had a profound effect upon me and my career, setting in motion a series of events that would make me, in many respects, a better physician and a better leader. I couldn't see that at the time.

As events unfolded over the next months and years, however, I was able to more clearly understand the various aspects of practicing in a highly competitive environment.

Then, though, I suddenly had to worry about a variety of factors, including (in no particular order): paying for my new house, calculating and executing the payout for my partner's death benefits, health insurance for my practice and my family, where the money was coming from in the practice, how much money was going out of the practice, how we were paying our employees, how we were managing our employees, how we were going to expand our business to absorb the loss of our great mentor and rainmaker, and, most importantly, how I, a young surgeon in the highly competitive Upper East Side of Manhattan, was going to build a practice and provide quality care to a highly sophisticated and demanding set of patients...the kind of care that I had always believed in and strived to provide for my patients.

In the following sections, we will explore a variety of these issues, providing real examples and tools that you can use in your own practice. Section 1 will review the "sharp" edge of the medical "business" including the language and tools required to succeed. By "sharp," I mean specific, often mathematical, tools that are required to understand the finances of a medical practice. These are the numbers you need to know, and without a basic understanding of them, you cannot even open your doors. Section 2 will address the "smooth" edge of building and maintaining a successful practice in an environment where it is becoming increasingly difficult to retain the loyalty of patients and referring physicians. By "smooth," I mean to connote a softer science. This section contains tools that you can use to manage the non-financial aspects of your practice. It would be a mistake to give this section short shrift. Without practicing excellence with a "smooth edge," there will be no finances with which to practice the "sharp edge." Finally, Section 3 will demonstrate what excellence with an edge looks like, by following the course of a single patient encounter through three sets of eyes: those of the referring physician, the staff, and the patient.

Practicing excellence with an edge will provide growth and stability for your practice, and provide the means and the time to focus on what you do best—provide excellent care to your patients.

SECTION 1
THE "SHARP"
edge
—LANGUAGE AND TOOLS TO EXCEL

In order to excel in today's competitive practice environment, you need to possess at least a basic understanding of the business of medicine and of the numbers that can make or break you. While it may be tempting to leave this to your accountant or office manager, it is clear that you can compete effectively—and make sound decisions—only by having a realistic and up-to-date financial picture of your practice.

In this section, we'll review the specific metrics you need to track in order to run a profitable medical practice and tools you can use today to help manage your accounts receivable. We will learn some of the language common to decision makers in all industries, and remove the mystery from financial concepts that determine whether any business (including yours) will thrive or fail. Finally, we'll go step-by-step through the development of a simple business plan that will help you evaluate the financial viability of a project (new hire, program, or equipment), giving you the credibility you need to get your next great idea funded.

CHAPTER 2

NUMBERS YOU MUST KNOW

· · · · · · · · · · ·

It was not long after my partner's death that his accountant called to discuss the execution of our partnership agreement, which delineated the payment to the estate of a deceased partner. Now, of course, as "the big guy" had been our practice's managing partner, his personal accountant was also our practice's accountant.

This led to an interesting potential conflict of interest, a discussion of which is beyond the scope of this book. Suffice it to say that this individual had intricate knowledge of the financial workings of our practice (much more than any of the remaining partners did). Fortunately for us, he was an honorable man and served as an honest broker, but it is easy to see how this could have been a problem in an adversarial relationship.

The main component of the money due my partner's estate was based upon the practice's outstanding accounts receivable, or A/R (money owed the practice). It seemed to me that I needed to delve into the world of A/R in order to ensure that the ultimate outcome of the accountant's analysis, and the resulting payout, was fair to both the estate and to the ongoing practice.

This exercise led me to ask a series of questions that I believe every physician must ask him or herself. To come up with accurate answers, it is critical to be familiar with at least some of the basic tools that people in all businesses use to get there.

My questions were these:
- Are we getting paid for our work?
- How much are we getting paid?
- How long does it take to get paid for the work we do, and what does that delay cost?
- How should we be tracking this?
- Is this something that I need to pay attention to other than in a time of crisis?

The answer to the last question is unequivocally yes.

Accounts receivable management is a potentially highly complex undertaking that virtually any and every business uses to varying degrees. Particularly in the medical field, where third-party and government payers abound, it can be extremely difficult to accurately track every penny that's owed you for the hard work and great care that you have provided.

Even within healthcare, certain physician organizations and practices will vary the sophistication with which they manage their A/R based on their size and complexity, as well as the nature of their contractual relationships with a variety of third-party payers.

> **There are certain features of accounts receivable management, however, that every single physician, whether in solo practice or employed by a large organization, must track and fully understand.**

Without knowledge of these basic concepts, you will never be in a position to understand the value (in monetary terms) of the services that you provide, both to your patients and to your organization.

How many of you know a doctor who seems angry all the time? He complains to anyone who will listen that he works more for less. However, his anger is almost certainly a manifestation of anxiety about the unknown. Knowledge of A/R management will allow you to better predict your income over a period of time and go a long way towards assuaging anxiety (and anger).

There are several specific metrics by which all medical practices (including yours, whether you know it or not) measure their productivity.

These metrics are:
- charges
- RVUs
- receipts
- accounts receivable
- days in accounts receivable
- charge lag
- denials

Intimate knowledge and tracking of these metrics are necessary, and usually sufficient, to ensure an appropriate revenue stream into the practice. In fact, one-page "dashboard"-type reports can be easily created to help track some or all of these measures. At a glance, you can get a snapshot of your practice's current financial picture.

Figure 2.1: Simple Dashboard Report

Physician Activity Report				January 1, 2010 - September 30, 2010					
Gross Charges	Jan $115,740	Feb $138,020	Mar $72,550	Apr $108,400	May $131,950	Jun $76,100	Jul $171,400	Aug $84,539	Sept $125,100	YTD $1,023,799
Net Receipts	Jan $21,221	Feb $45,353	Mar $39,129	Apr $30,224	May $47,670	Jun $47,877	Jul $33,795	Aug $36,162	Sept $26,275	YTD $327,706
RVUs	Jan 427.29	Feb 473.97	Mar 215.12	Apr 342.05	May 460.27	Jun 253.54	Jul 513.16	Aug 206.02	Sept 406.73	YTD 3,298.15
Days in A/R	Jan 62	Feb 59	Mar 60	Apr 58	May 63	Jun 63	Jul 67	Aug 71	Sept 73	CURRENT 73
Charge Lag	Jan 5	Feb 5	Mar 9	Apr 4	May 12	Jun 5	Jul 8	Aug 6	Sept 4	YTD (AVG) 6.4

This simple dashboard report can be created on a monthly basis by anyone with a computer. I used just such a report early on in my practice.

Larger organizations will often use more sophisticated software to create automated, interactive reports, like the one in Figure 2.2.

Figure 2.2: More Sophisticated Dashboard Report

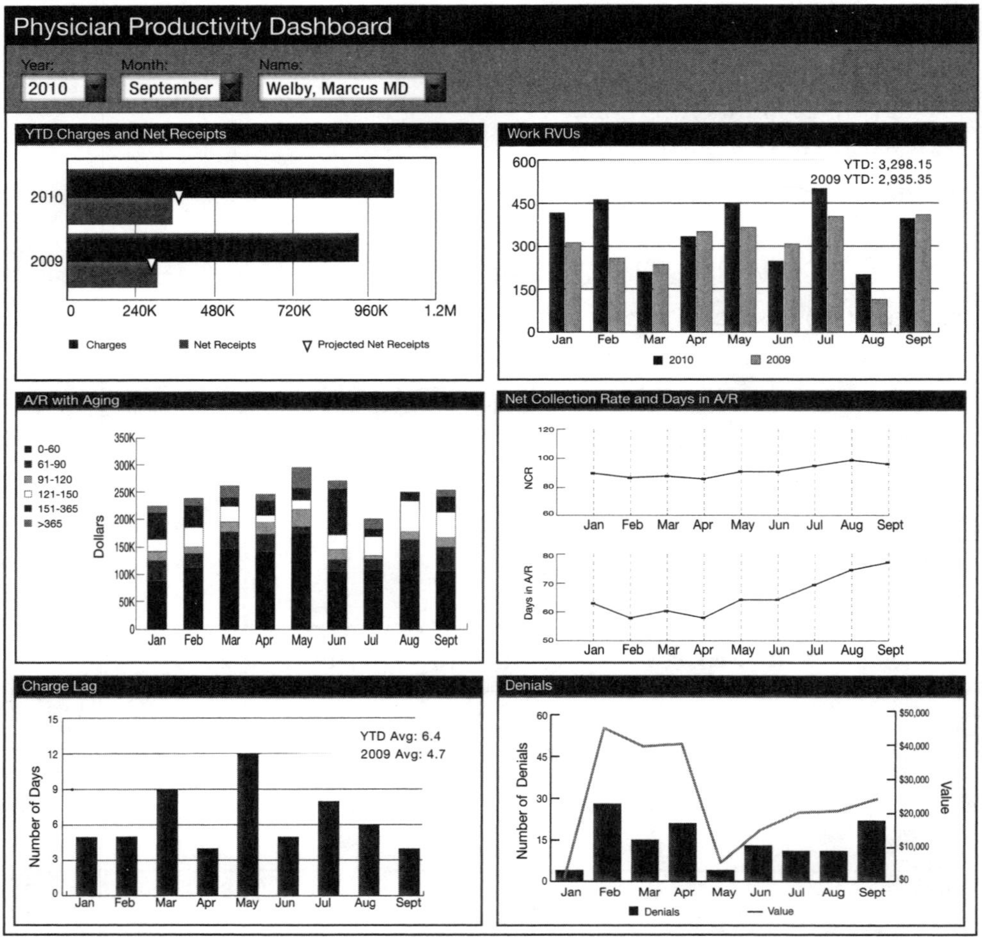

With a quick glance at the middle graphs, you can easily spot a trend of rising days in A/R, suggesting a potential problem that needs to be reviewed.

Dashboards like this allow the physician or manager to drill down into one or more of the components to see monthly or even daily values and evaluate issues such as this.

Let's examine each of these metrics separately.

Charges

In their simplest form, charges are the amount of money that you bill for the services that you provide. While one might think this would be quite straightforward, there are actually a number of different ways to review your charges, which have implications on your A/R management. The easiest number to understand is gross charges. Gross charges are the total dollar amount of charges created when your full fee schedule is applied to each of the services you provide.

Put another way, it is the total dollar value of the work that you do in a perfect world. Clearly it is not a perfect world, which is why you have accounts receivable in the first place. Many billing software programs used by physicians list gross charges in their basic A/R analysis, so this is probably a metric with which you are already familiar.

To me, the intimate pairing of gross charges with receipts is a mistake leading to a tremendous amount of frustration and misunderstanding. The discrepancy is often so large as to be downright depressing. But as it is very likely to be a part of any dashboard, I have included it in Figures 2.1 and 2.2.

Imagine, for a moment, that you have a high proportion of your practice that has Medicare as their insurance carrier. If you live in a competitive environment, such as a big city, it is likely that your fee schedule is considerably higher than that which you know Medicare will allow. A higher fee schedule is, of course, legal—and even desirable—because it is your hope that many patients will pay you or have insurance plans that will pay you at much higher rates than will Medicare.

As an aside, you must remember that every patient must be billed at the same amount, for the same level of service, regardless of his method of payment. This mandate comes from interstate commerce laws that would seem to have no bearing on medical billing. So there is no value to lowering your fee schedule to reflect Medicare rates (nor can you bill Medicare patients at a level less than your standard fee schedule). Having said that, it is clear that the only money that you will receive, ultimately, will be determined at Medicare rates in this particular instance.

For example: If you charge $100 for a service and you know Medicare pays only $27, there is a $73 differential from what you are charging to what you know you are going to receive. Multiply this out hundreds of times, and apply it across multiple payer systems with differing reimbursement rates, and you can easily see why your gross charges have little bearing on real-life expectations of payment. This is demonstrated in the Totals column in Figure 2.1, where the difference between Gross Charges and Net Receipts is $696,093.

Physician Activity Report				January 1, 2010 - September 30, 2010					
Gross Charges	Jan $115,740	Feb $138,020	Mar $72,550	Apr $108,400	May $131,950	Jun $76,100	Jul $171,400	Aug $84,539	Sept $125,100	**YTD $1,023,799**
Net Receipts	Jan $21,221	Feb $45,353	Mar $39,129	Apr $30,224	May $47,670	Jun $47,877	Jul $33,795	Aug $36,162	Sept $26,275	**YTD $327,706**

This is why, by itself, using gross charges as a metric is of limited value. Following this number over time, however, can give you a sense of the volume and quality of the work you are doing. Trends will emerge that can be useful for practice management.

RVUs

Many physician groups, particularly large and multi-specialty groups, use relative value units (RVUs) in order to track physician productivity. This metric can be useful to managers of large groups because it is a way of reliably comparing the productivity of doctors across a variety of different specialties. It is imperative for the individual physician to understand and track his or her RVUs, as well, for a variety of reasons I will touch upon below.

Some of you may find the history of the RVU system fascinating (many more of you may not), and I encourage you to read about it. Briefly, the Health Care Financing Administration (now called the Centers for Medicare and Medicaid Services) introduced the RVU system in 1992 as a method of tracking payments from Medicare for physician work. The scale attempts to quantify the relative value of any given CPT code based on a number of factors, about 55 percent of which is based upon the complexity and time value of the work performed by the physician. Practice factors, which attempt to compensate for the expenses of the practice (such as labor, materials, and supplies), make up most of the rest of this value. There is also a malpractice expense factor built into the code.

Medicare payments for a service are derived by multiplying the RVUs for that CPT code by a factor that is determined by Congress on an annual basis. In 2010, the multiplier is 36.0846 dollars. Besides Medicare, almost all insurance carriers calculate payments to physicians based on the RVU scale. As you can imagine, the lobbying efforts of all of the medical specialties to maximize the RVU values of their own codes—at the expense of others—is fierce.

While the debate continues to rage on regarding the fairness of the current RVU scale, there is quite a bit of reproducibility across the years and across various specialties. Individual practices certainly can use the total number of RVUs billed in any given period to serve as a useful measure of productivity.

As with many other metrics, tracking the *trend* in RVUs is an extremely useful method of following physician productivity across various time periods. For example, an examination of Figure 2.1 shows a dramatic drop in production in August, as measured in both RVU and gross charges. However, simple investigation revealed that the physician in question was on vacation for ten days that month, so no cause for alarm.

Physician Activity Report			
July 1, 2010 - September 30, 2010			
Gross Charges	Jul $171,400	Aug $84,539	Sept $125,100
RVUs	Jul 513.16	Aug 206.02	Sept 406.73

You should know that most physician organizations and, importantly, insurance companies and hospitals track RVUs religiously. Any negotiation with outside entities will almost always have relative value units as a part of that negotiation. For example, medical practices seeking to merge will use RVUs as an indicator of the relative productivity of the merging groups. In surgical and procedural specialties, knowledge of your RVUs is a critical piece of information that allows you to effectively negotiate deals with hospitals or other agencies.

I once worked with a group of general surgeons who were extremely busy, but who weren't being compensated at a level that seemed commensurate with their clinical activities. Simple tracking of their RVUs revealed that they were, indeed, doing a high volume of work. Their receipts were low because they were doing mostly Medicaid work, but the hospital was doing a booming business. This knowledge enabled the group to negotiate a very favorable deal with the hospital, in which everyone could benefit from the excellent care they were providing to a group of underserved patients.

Another way that RVUs can be used in managing your practice is to look at the kinds of visits or procedures you are performing. For example, if you are a gastroenterologist with x-ray capabilities, you may have the ability to do barium enemas or colonoscopies. Colonoscopy (CPT code 45378) has an RVU assignment of 10.37. Barium enema (CPT code 74270) is 3.93 RVUs. Given that they both take about the same amount of time, and that colonoscopy has the potential to be therapeutic and is a more sensitive diagnostic tool, which procedure would you choose to increase?

Receipts

Receipts are fairly simple. Receipts are clear. Receipts are good. Receipts are necessary. Receipts are quite simply the amount of money that you actually get for the services that you provide. They allow you to pay your bills, to pay your employees, and to pay yourself at the end of the day. We typically think of receipts as being gross receipts, which is the total dollar value of the money that comes in, but this can be a bit misleading. The number we are more interested in is net receipts, which are gross receipts minus refunds.

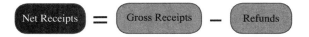

Many practices will attempt (correctly) to collect some or all of the money owed them directly from their patients. This can take the form of a "time of service" payment or a deposit on future services and is useful for a practice's cash flow. It is much easier to collect money at or prior to the time of service than it is to chase people down long after a service has been provided.

It is possible that the money collected directly from a patient plus the money paid by the insurance company may exceed your total charge for that service. For example, if you charge $100 for a service, collect $50 as a time of service payment or deposit directly from the patient, and the insurance company ultimately pays $70 for that service, your receipts will be $120. You will be required (by law and by ethics) to refund $20 to the patient. Sometimes through negotiated settlements with the insurance companies, you will be required to refund more.

Clearly, in this setting, you have not earned $120, and yet your gross receipts reflect that you have. This is not particularly useful, which is why we should use the more specific parameter, net receipts, which reflects your total receipts minus refunds. This is the true measure of the dollar intake of a physician practice.

It should be intuitively obvious that if there were a single number that a physician or physician practice should know, it is net receipts. Failure to follow this metric will result in certain disaster.

Like any household (but apparently unlike the government), a practice can't spend more than it brings in. Net receipts is the pure measure of what you "bring in."

Accounts Receivable

Conceptually, accounts receivable can be viewed as money you are still owed for services you have already provided. Formulaically, A/R is simply calculated as:

$$\text{Accounts Receivable} = \text{Charges} - \text{Receipts}$$

It is the management of this number that distinguishes good management from poor, successful businesses from failed, and sane physicians from lunatics.

Speaking of lunatics, when we last left off, I was attempting to calculate and execute the payout for my recently departed partner. A/R was the linchpin of the calculated settlement. The formula was simple enough. It was based on a percentage of the total A/R of the practice.

This formula had been handed down through generations of the practice. It was purported to have been based on a historical norm, but I remain convinced to this day that it was what venture capitalists call "blue sky," which essentially means the numbers were plucked from thin air. It was the shock value of the magnitude of the number in this instance that drove me to learn about A/R management. I was determined never to be caught so unaware again.

Here was the problem. The accounts receivable calculation came from every charge and every receipt from the beginning of time (or at least from the beginning of our computerized billing system, approximately eight years earlier). My first thought was, *There is no way that we're expecting to collect anywhere near the projected return on these accounts receivable.*

Intuitively, I knew this to be the case. Some of these accounts were $26 balances from patients, long since deceased (of old age, of course), for whom we had cared seven years earlier. I hoped we weren't continuing to try to collect on those accounts. It certainly wasn't worth the valuable time of our billing staff. I'm not even certain it was worth the cost of the envelopes and stamps required to dun those accounts.

It turned out that my intuition was correct...and what I had guessed had been long worked out in healthcare and every other industry since the beginning of time. A/R management begins with the concept of "the time value of money." This concept says that with every tick of the clock, your money, in someone else's pocket, declines in value.

For traditional industries, a good rule of thumb is that the value of a dollar, uncollected at two months, has declined by ten percent. By six months, that dollar is worth half. At a year, the decline accelerates, so that by two years, the value of that dollar is less than a nickel!

It is widely believed that the decline of a healthcare receivable dollar is much steeper. There are a variety of explanations for this, not the least important of which is the relative inexperience of doctors in managing our financial and business affairs (one of the raisons d'être of this book).

And so, I took these accounts receivables to be looked at by a business called a "factor." A factor is someone who purchases businesses' accounts receivable for a discount and then assumes the burden of collection. I was nearly laughed out of the room.

He barely had to look at the accounts to know that most of it was going to be uncollectible. Also, he explained, doctors are notorious "soft touches"; we went into medicine to help people. We are uncomfortable with the aggressive pursuit of the collection of old debts. Most factors won't even talk to doctors.

Before moving on to the next section on aging of accounts receivable, a word about the formula itself. You will recall that we have no reasonable expectation, in many cases, that we will receive payment for our full charge. In many of these situations, we have the ability to predict with real accuracy how much money we can anticipate from certain charges. Mostly, these fall into the realm of contractual obligations. Examples of this are Medicare fees and negotiated "in-network" fees for insurance panels.

So a more useful parameter to follow, rather than gross A/R, is net accounts receivable, which is calculated by accounts receivable minus contractual allowances. In long form, net accounts receivable are charges minus contractual allowances minus receipts.

$$\text{Net A/R} = \text{Charges} - \text{Contractual Allowances} - \text{Receipts}$$

This is the number off of which a practice should begin to work in order to attempt to maximize its collections. It is a truer representation of what you "expect" to collect, particularly when evaluating current patients. Many billing programs allow this calculation to be automated. I highly recommend this.

Aging of Accounts Receivable

As we saw earlier, the longer a debt is outstanding to you, the less valuable that debt becomes. Nowhere is this more true than in your medical practice's accounts receivable.

That's why management of the aging of your accounts receivable is a critical part of ensuring that you are well-compensated for your services.

In its simplest form, A/R management would seem relatively easy. You perform a service on day zero and submit a bill for that service. You check daily to see the status of that bill and whether or not you've been paid. When payment arrives you are able to reduce your accounts receivable by that amount and look to the patient or secondary insurance company for the balance.

In practice, however, it is much more complex than that. Depending on the size of your practice and whether or not you are attached to a huge multi-specialty practice or hospital, the degree of sophistication with which your receivables are managed is very variable.

Additionally, most of you are not at day zero in your practice and have accounts receivable that have already aged significantly. For you, A/R management has two major components. First, old accounts must be "cleaned up." Next, a management program for your current A/R must be put into place.

So, looking at the A/R in my practice, which consisted of eight years of accounts, it was clear that we had no system of easily understanding the true value of this asset (more on assets later) or of predicting how much of this figure we were likely to collect; therefore, its only value as a tool for us was to be able to calculate the enormous dollar figure that we owed our deceased partner's estate. Unfortunately for us, our A/R was unrealistically inflated because we had not tightly managed it over the years.

So I set out to clean up our old A/R. The first and easiest task was to get a bird's-eye view of the "aging." This means looking at the dollar amount of the accounts receivable broken down by the date of service. Each account was placed in a certain "bucket," defined by how many days it had been since the service was provided. In most medical practices, those buckets are as follows: 0-60 days, 61-90 days, 91-120 days, 121-150 days, 151-365 days, and more than 365 days.

Figure 2.3: Aging of Accounts Receivable: Small Group Practice

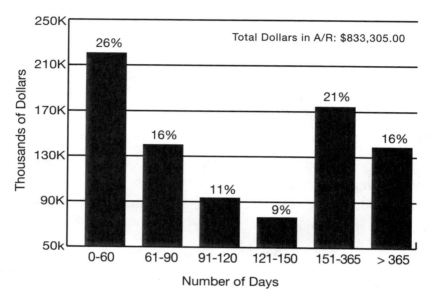

In this example of A/R aging for a small group practice, the doctors have a big problem with old accounts.

In a well-managed practice, the last two buckets will be very low. Take a look at this next example of how A/R is distributed at this large multi-specialty practice. Even this efficient group has some work to do on its A/R in the 151-365 bucket.

Figure 2.4: Aging of Accounts Receivable: Large Multi-specialty Practice

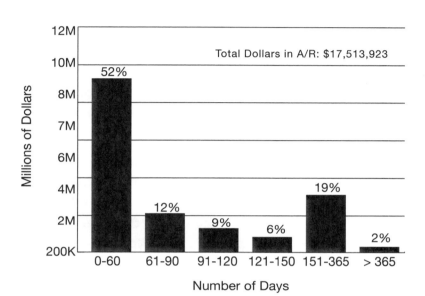

Alternatively, many people will simply look at the percentage of their A/R that is more than 120 days old and track that number. Obviously, the smaller the number, the more efficient your organization is at collecting. You'll note that 365 days is the inner limit of the last bucket. Beyond that, there seems to be very little value at further classifying time frames. This should tell you something right off the bat about the time value of money (see above).

In the clean-up phase of our operation, we looked at every account that was more than 365 days old. Many of them were for a dollar amount that was so low that we were actually losing money by generating statements to those people. Remember, it costs at least several dollars to send a single statement when labor, stamps, envelopes, and paper are accounted for.

Some estimates of the average cost of an attempt to collect any account over six months old exceed $30. When you multiply the cost of collections for these old accounts by the number of years you do this, you are clearly losing money.

Write Off Small Old Accounts and Evaluate Large Ones

So the first task in cleaning up a book of accounts receivable is to write off any and all accounts that are simply not worth pursuing because they are too old and too small. This will immediately have the effect of reducing your accounts receivable and reducing the percentage of the accounts receivable that is greater than 120 days.

The next task is to look at the larger accounts and evaluate them individually to see whether it is reasonable that any payment is forthcoming. It is wise to be fairly aggressive at writing off these accounts as well. You will find that many of them fall into a variety of categories that can be written off quickly.

For example, you will likely find that many of these accounts will be uncollectible due to failure of timely filing.

Most insurance payers require charges to be filed, or appeals to be addressed, within a defined time frame (usually 90 days). You are also likely to find that many unpaid claims were denied because the proper referral wasn't obtained prior to the service being provided. Many of these accounts will still be in receivables due to a variety of other denials (more about denials later).

In evaluating these denials, many of your accounts will be deemed absolutely unrecoverable. Write them off.

Review Other Accounts on a Case-by-Case Basis

After you have written off old accounts and evaluated larger accounts, the next step is to consider negotiating some of the A/R that remain, in order to collect more money sooner. You will no doubt find that many of these patients and their accounts will be on payment plans. I can't tell you how many patients we found with balances of over $1,000 who were paying at a rate of $15 a month.

At that rate, it would take more than five-and-a-half years to repay the debt. Those accounts warrant a negotiation. I would much rather have $500 or even $300 in my pocket today than the prospect of $15 a month for five-and-a-half years. There are formulas that are readily available to help make that value calculation. (Google "net present value" to get started.)

Finally, there will be a group of patients that you just have to decide how aggressively you want to pursue. This will have to be done on a case-by-case basis. In doing this, you will learn just how much of a "soft touch" you really are.

> **However, I strongly recommend that you aggressively pursue the accounts of those patients who have received a check from the insurance company for your services, cashed the check, but have refused to pay you.**

I know of very few things that anger physicians more than this, and it happens all the time.

Ultimately, a decision has to be made on how to deal with the remainder of your accounts. This can be done on a case-by-case basis, but, again, in order to effectively move forward, one has to be brutally honest in one's appraisal of the value of these accounts. Remember, any account that remains on the books, remains on the books, and you'll have to deal with it again and again and again, each time you perform such an exercise.

Going forward, it is much better to ensure your accounts do not get to this point. In the case of my practice, we had left tens, if not hundreds, of thousands of dollars on the table prior to our "awakening." Thinking about it even now makes me cringe.

It is worth remembering that capturing income is not just about profitability. By ensuring your practice is compensated accurately for care provided, you ensure that you will have the resources necessary to provide quality care to patients in the years to come; to retain high-performing employees who exceed patient expectations; to grow the practice so that patients have timely access; and to invest in the technology and resources your physicians need to ensure quality clinical outcomes. Nothing is more important than this in our work.

Days in Accounts Receivable

Once you have dealt with old A/R, the management phase (which never ends) can be addressed in earnest. Remember that as you are performing this exercise every day, accounts are moving from one bucket into the next as accounts continue to age. A single number that can be used very effectively by every physician is called Days in Accounts Receivable.

> **I believe that following the trend of this one metric is enough for most practitioners to assess the ongoing efficiency of their billing and collections and alert physicians to problems as they arise.**

There are a number of formulas that can be used to calculate days in accounts receivable. The most basic formula is:

$$\text{Days in A/R} = \text{Net Accounts Receivable} \div \text{Average Daily Receipts}$$

Average daily receipts can be taken by dividing monthly receipts by 30, quarterly receipts by 90, or annual receipts by 365. I recommend using 90 days to calculate average daily receipts because it is a long enough period to be meaningful and a short enough one to allow trends to be easily spotted.

Many larger practices and healthcare organizations use the following formula:

$$\text{Days in A/R} = \text{Gross Accounts Receivable} \div \text{Average Daily Gross Charges}$$

While this method of calculating days in A/R may be less precise than the formula noted above—remember that gross A/R and gross charges are often unrealistically inflated—it is easier to measure across various practice types and organizations. That is why this is the preferred formula for benchmarking by many industry groups, including the Medical Group Management Association (MGMA) and the Association of American Medical Colleges (AAMC).

In either case, the numerical result is an indication of the average number of days it takes to collect for a service. While the absolute number is itself important (as it provides a snapshot of the general efficiency of your billing operation *at that moment in time*), it is the *trend* in days in A/R that will prove to be more useful to you as a practitioner. Using this parameter on your monthly dashboard allows you to quickly spot disturbing patterns. If you see a spike in your days in A/R, it can alert you to drill deeper to find the source. (You can contact the MGMA for specialty- and practice-type benchmarks for days in A/R.)

Figure 2.5: Days in A/R

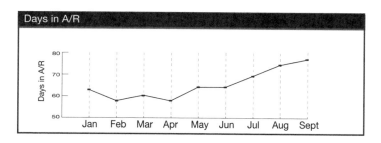

In this graph, the upward trend in A/R days demonstrates a problem that needs to be investigated. Now.

You may think that tracking an arcane metric such as days in accounts receivable is a purely academic exercise in accounting that has no real bearing on your day-to-day life, but actually, following this trend will allow you to quickly and accurately assess the ongoing efficiency of your entire billing operation (whether that consists of your spouse, a few people, or an entire office of billing personnel).

And it translates into real money. For example, if your annual net receipts are about $600,000, making your average daily receipts about $1,650, a reduction of just four days in A/R puts $6,600 in your pocket. This is only a one-time gain, but I'll take it!

As Quint Studer points out in his book *Straight A Leadership: Alignment, Action, Accountability*, we can learn a lot from hospital chief financial officers (CFOs). While they often get a bad rap for "penny pinching," it is really their ability to develop, measure, and hold others accountable to specific, objective goals that keeps hospitals viable. By keeping a close watch on financial variances, they are quick to respond to changes in organizational performance before problems get out of control and impact the organization's ability to meet its mission.

In fact, as Studer notes, if you ask most CFOs how many days of cash collections they must fall behind before they start to take action (e.g., ask questions to dig deeper), the answer is nearly always "three to five days." Can you say the same about your practice?

Charge Lag

This one is simple. Charge lag is the average difference between the date of service and the date that you post a charge. It seems silly to even mention, but you can't collect on a bill you haven't posted. In many practices, physicians and their staff average days, if not weeks, before posting their charges. Tracking this number on a regular basis can help you manage your billing operation much more effectively. No need to look for practice benchmarks here. Your goal should be zero. The same math that we saw for days in A/R applies here.

Denials

So now that you have committed to posting your charges in a timely fashion, it is time to remember a simple truth in A/R management: "Clean claims get paid." Given the complexity of the third-party reimbursement system in medicine, it is amazing that we get paid at all.

In order for the government (Medicare or Medicaid) or any insurance company to process an insurance claim for a medical service, every single piece of information in the claim must be perfectly accurate. Failure to do exactly what is asked will lead to "denials."

These denials can take many forms and can be extremely costly to your medical practice. It is estimated that 10 to 15 percent of all healthcare claims are delayed or denied due to errors. I don't know about you, but it seems to me that the real percentage is much higher. Up to 50 percent of denied claims are never re-filed[4], meaning that by attrition, doctors' offices are giving away money often due to simple mistakes. This made up a large part of the money my practice had "lost" over the years.

The tragedy of all of this is that at least 90 percent of denials are preventable. My purpose here is not to list the various types of denials and edits that you encounter on a daily basis. However, tracking the absolute number and/or the dollar value of your denials on a regular basis can give you an ongoing measure of the efficiency of your billing operation and alert you to problems before they become too great.

Again, the best way to manage denials is to prevent them in the first place by submitting clean claims that have been appropriately coded and "scrubbed" for errors. Most billing software programs have optional claims scrubbing modules, and many external services can assist you in this function. I strongly urge you to consider this.

Who's in Charge of This Stuff?

The level at which medical practices manage and use these financial tools varies greatly depending on the size and scope of the practice. In individual practices, physicians may use simpler tools and manage this aspect of the practice themselves, ask a spouse to handle it, or delegate it to a single employee. On the other end of the spectrum—in large, multi-specialty groups—a whole office full of people may use very sophisticated financial management software. Or it might be outsourced.

In any case, regardless of who manages the financial health of your practice, it is critical to ensure proper oversight, clear goals, frequent performance reviews, and accountability. And you, the doctor, must have a set of metrics—a dashboard of some sort—that you regularly review to ensure that your practice is moving in the right direction. This is not optional.

Key Learning Points: Numbers You MUST Know

1. Understand how much your practice is getting paid for its work, how long it takes to get paid, what payment delays cost, and how to track these numbers on an ongoing basis.

2. The metrics you need to understand and track are charges, RVUs, receipts, accounts receivable (A/R), days in accounts receivable, charge lag, and denials.

3. Use a one-page "dashboard" report to keep current on the metrics above.

4. To manage A/R effectively, you will need to first "clean up" old accounts by writing them off, evaluate large accounts, and negotiate payment for some accounts to collect more money sooner.

5. Follow this one trend—Days in Accounts Receivable.

6. Who manages these financial metrics depends on the size, scope, and sophistication of the practice.

7. You must provide oversight. The buck stops with you.

CHAPTER 3
NUMBERS YOU SHOULD KNOW
(EVERYONE ELSE DOES)

· · · · · · · · · · ·

In the weeks and months after I took over the management of the practice, I wrote—or, to be more accurate, signed—a lot of checks. I actually thought I was pretty cool because I used one of those big, leather-bound checkbooks with three checks on a page and carbon backups so that each check could be looked at from our own records. It had one of those big cardboard blocks that you would put behind the active page so that you weren't damaging the carbon copies of the next set of checks. What could be more professional than this?

I was signing checks to the employees.
I was signing checks to the grocery store.
To the electrician. To the plumber. To the lawyer.
To the accountant. To myriad different "vendors."

One day I was signing a fairly sizeable check to, of all things, our health insurance plan, and I asked the officer manager two questions that, although seemingly innocuous, set off a series of events that really demonstrated the dearth of my management knowledge.

The first question was, "Do we have enough money in the bank to cover this check?" The second was, "What did we spend on insurance last year?" Unfortunately, the office manager shrugged and couldn't easily answer either question.

By pursuing the answers to these questions, I learned to ask a series of questions that every other business asks itself on a regular basis. My questions were these:

- What is our cash position?
- What is our business's financial health?
- What does it cost to keep our doors open?
- What does it cost to take care of patients?
- And at the end of this, are we making a profit?

Also, what are those reports that my accountant keeps sending us? Are these useful to me, in any real sense? Once again, the answer to that last question is unequivocally yes.

In this chapter we will explore the universal concepts of basic accounting, which are critical to the ability of a physician to communicate with people at all levels of all businesses in all industries.

Some of the concepts we will discuss include:
- cash basis versus accrual basis accounting
- the chart of accounts
- assets and liabilities
- financial statements
- the nature of costs and revenues

We'll look at examples from an institutional perspective (medical school and/or hospital) as well as from the practice side (private and academic). I apologize in advance for the material in this chapter. It's true that even accountants find accounting boring! However, ignore these concepts at your own peril.

Cash Basis Versus Accrual Basis Accounting

I am not an accountant. Nor do I play one on TV. But I, along with every other human being on the planet, use accounting every day.

There are two basic methods of accounting for revenues and expenses that are used by most businesses. The first and simplest is called "cash basis" accounting. In its basic form, cash basis accounting recognizes transactions, revenues, and expenses when money changes hands.

In a medical practice, this means that revenues (mostly receipts) are put on the books when the money comes in. If you perform a service for a patient in January and get paid in May, it is in May when the revenue is booked in cash basis accounting. Similarly, when you pay your plumber in July for work done in June, it is July when the expense is incurred.

In "accrual basis" accounting, the opposite is true. Revenue is recognized when services are provided. Expenses are placed on the books when resources are consumed, regardless of when the money actually changes hands.

While there are a variety of arguments for one method of accounting versus the other—involving tax reporting requirements, financial planning and control, contractual issues, and other issues—the overwhelming majority of medical practices operate on the cash basis. Good thing, too, because for us doctors, it is much easier to understand.

There are, of course, small but important nuances that we must heed. Take, for example, my initial question: Do we have enough money in the bank to cover this check? The answer was not so readily available. My first instinct was to call the bank. Easy enough. Call the bank. What's my balance? Done, right?

Actually, no. The problem is that while there was clearly enough money to cover this check in the bank at that moment, the account officer couldn't take into account the fact that there were numerous other checks that I had already written and signed, but that had not, necessarily, been cleared at the bank. These "checks in transit" had the ability to throw off my bank balance enough to create the possibility of an overdraft.

A better way to get a true picture of available funds would be to "reconcile" the checkbook, which would require a daily accounting of which checks had been cleared by the bank and which had not. Additionally, we'd need to know and account for the daily cash deposits into the bank to maintain an accurate accounting of our bank balance. This is a labor-intensive process, but one that is absolutely critical to understand in order to answer my question about our cash position. I am fairly certain that you or a member of your household does this at home on a (semi) regular basis.

While it was relatively new on the scene at that time, software that will manage exactly this type of exercise is now readily available and almost ubiquitous. In addition to banks' proprietary software, third-party products such as QuickBooks and Microsoft Money make this process much more manageable. Many programs will even automatically download transactions from your financial institutions and reconcile your checkbook on a real-time basis.

Chart of Accounts

The answer to my second question (What did we spend on insurance last year?) required an enormous amount of effort. In order to figure this out, the office manager had to thumb through boxes and boxes of the carbon copies of checks that I described to you earlier. Even then, we were not entirely certain that the answer was accurate.

QuickBooks Pro, which was my financial software of choice, again ultimately resolved this issue. I learned that every accounting system is organized into a "chart of accounts," which essentially serves to identify and classify various types of revenues and expenses.

On the revenue side of a medical practice, it's really quite simple because the overwhelming majority of revenue comes from receipts for patient care. More complicated medical practices, with managed care contracts and/or research components, may have a more complicated revenue stream.

On the expense side, however, we all seem to spend money on essentially the same things. The chart of accounts, which can be quite simple or quite complex, allows you to categorize the expenses and follow them from time period to time period.

One of the beautiful things about these third-party software programs is that they create sample charts of accounts for a variety of different industries, including medical practices.

Figure 3.1: Sample Chart of Accounts

Account	Type	Account	Type
Owner's Capital	Equity	Petty Cash	Expense
Draws	Equity	Postage and Delivery	Expense
Investments	Equity	Printing and Reproduction	Expense
Retained Earnings	Equity	Professional Development	Expense
Fee Refunds	Income	Professional Fees	Expense
Fees	Income	Accounting	Expense
Consultation	Income	Consulting	Expense
Patient Fees	Income	Legal Fees	Expense
Investment Income	Income	Reference Materials	Expense
Legal Chart Reviews	Income	Rent	Expense
Rental Income	Income	Repairs	Expense
Research Grants	Income	Building Repairs	Expense
Advertising Expense	Expense	Computer Repairs	Expense
Amortization Expense	Expense	Equipment Repairs	Expense
Automobile Expense	Expense	Supplies	Expense
Bank Service Charges	Expense	Marketing	Expense
Cash Discounts	Expense	Medical	Expense
Computer	Expense	Office	Expense
Contract Labor	Expense	Taxes	Expense
Contributions	Expense	Federal	Expense
Depreciation Expense	Expense	Local	Expense
Dictations Service	Expense	Property	Expense
Dues and Subscriptions	Expense	State	Expense
Equipment Rental	Expense	Telephone	Expense
Insurance	Expense	Travel & Ent	Expense
Disability Insurance	Expense	Entertainment	Expense
Liability Insurance	Expense	Meals	Expense
Malpractice Insurance	Expense	Travel	Expense
Medical Insurance	Expense	Utilities	Expense
Work Comp	Expense	Gas & Electric	Expense
Interest Expense	Expense	Water	Expense
Finance Charge	Expense	Waste Disposal	Expense
Loan Interest	Expense	Interest Income	Other Income
Mortgage	Expense	Other Income	Other Income
Laboratory Fees	Expense	Other Expenses	Other Expense
Laundry	Expense	Writeoff	Other Expense
Licenses and Permits	Expense		
Management	Expense		
Medical	Expense		
Office Supplies	Expense		
Payroll and Taxes	Expense		
Payroll	Expense		
Payroll Services	Expense		
Payroll Taxes	Expense		

In subsequent years, following the introduction of this software to my practice, I could tell you, to the penny, what we spent on groceries in the second quarter of any year. I could easily find out how that compared to the second quarter of any prior year, as well, to determine whether or not we were eating too much. This is equally true of the insurance data I was looking for, and, indeed, for any expenses that I wished to compare to any prior period. Once established, this kind of simple accounting system contains data that is readily mined to answer virtually all other questions regarding the financial makeup of your medical practice. We will explore some of these in subsequent sections of this chapter.

Assets and Liabilities

Now that you have established your cash position by understanding what your true bank balance is, we can take the next step in understanding the business's current financial position by looking at what accountants call a "balance sheet."

The balance sheet is probably the simplest of the financial statements that an accountant uses to determine the financial position of any entity, including a medical practice. It essentially has two columns, where, on one side, is listed all of the business's "assets," and on the other is listed its "liabilities." At any given time in a viable business's life, the two columns should "balance" out or be equivalent.

Figure 3.2: Sample Balance Sheet

Medical Practice			
Balance Sheet			
As of April 7, 2010			

ASSETS		LIABILITIES & EQUITY	
Current Assets		**Liabilities**	
Checking/Savings		Current Liabilities	
Cash Receipts	102,530.52	Line of Credit - 1	-357.54
Payroll Checking Account	130.04	Line of Credit - 2	-401,294.52
Research Fund Account	3,609.20		
Money Market	205,032.70	Total Current Liabilties	-401,652.06
Office Real Estate Account	37,358.00		
Operating Account	-104,334.09	Long-Term Liabilities	
Payroll Account	21,935.75	Capital Equipment Loan	-37,614.26
Savings Account	152,513.90		
Rollover Checking Account	39,118.73	Total Liabilities	-439,266.32
Total Checking/Savings	457,894.75	**Equity**	
Total Current Assets	457,894.75	Opening Bal Equity	-15,358.68
		Retained Earnings	1,051,777.52
Other Assets		Total Equity	1,036,418.84
Furniture and Equipment	139,257.77		
Total Other Assets	139,257.77		
TOTAL ASSETS	597,152.52	**TOTAL LIABILITIES & EQUITY**	597,152.52

Assets are those things that have positive value. Examples are cash in the bank, accounts receivable, stocks and bonds, real estate, furniture and equipment, and anything else that has monetary value. Remember that not all assets are necessarily equal. For example, as noted earlier, cash in hand is certainly much more readily available and usable than accounts receivables, which, while valuable, are much less liquid. In fact, in cash basis accounting, A/R doesn't even count as an asset on the balance sheet!

On the other side of the sheet are liabilities. Liabilities are anything with negative value. Examples of liabilities are accounts payable (or bills due), outstanding loans owed (such as bank loans or mortgages due), and money owed to employees. A side note: From a financial statement point of view, employees and other personnel are considered costs or liabilities. The smart business owner knows otherwise; in fact, good people are any business's best asset.

You must remember that a balance sheet is essentially a snapshot in time. It tells you only what is happening—what your financial position is—at the moment at which the balance sheet is created. The numbers on a balance sheet, in any given business, are likely to change on a daily, if not hourly, basis. When the numbers in the asset column are added up, they will equal the sum of the liabilities.

You are probably thinking, *How could that possibly be true? How can that always be the case?* The answer lies in the piece that I did not mention yet, which is "owners' equity." Owners' equity is what's left when the other assets and liabilities are all tallied. If the assets are greater than the liabilities, then the owners' equity is positive, meaning that if the business were to liquidate at that moment, the owners would walk away with something in their pockets.

On the other hand, if the liabilities exceed the assets, then the owners will have "negative equity," meaning that they will need to find a way to satisfy their creditors. However, balance sheets are not created on the day a business ends. They are typically created on a quarterly basis and provide a useful management tool for any physician to evaluate the current financial position of his or her practice.

Profit and Loss

The other main financial reporting instrument that your accountant sends on a quarterly and annual basis is called a "profit and loss statement" (or P&L). Unlike the balance sheet, which, as we showed, was essentially a snapshot in time, the P&L evaluates the financial activities of a practice over a period of time (either a quarter or a year).

Essentially, the P&L adds up all of the money spent during the period (costs) and subtracts that total from the money that came in over that same period (revenues). The result is "net income," also known as the "bottom line." A positive number is considered to be a profit, where a negative number is, unfortunately, a loss. An example of a simple P&L for a medical practice is in Figure 3.3.

Figure 3.3: Sample Profit and Loss Statement

Medical Practice
Profit and Loss Previous Year Comparison
1st Quarter 2010

	1 Q 2010	1 Q 2009	$ Change	% Change
Ordinary Income/Expense				
Income				
Cash	5,183	1,992	3,191	160%
Fees	1,120,938	1,162,332	-41,394	-4%
Int Income	2,462	465	1,997	429%
Total Income	1,128,583	1,164,789	-36,206	3%
Expense				
Advertising	588	476	112	24%
Automobile Expense	22,469	20,814	1,655	8%
Bank Service Charges	4,032	1,753	2,279	130%
Bldg. Maintenance	9,965	7,102	2,863	40%
Charity	0	45	-45	-100%
Computer Expense	2,480	2,320	160	7%
Dictation	700	1,103	-403	-37%
Dinner Meeting	667	1,008	-341	-34%
Electronic Equipment	975	325	650	200%
Goodwill	2,402	4,569	-2,167	-47%
Groceries	4,671	4,968	-297	-6%
Insurance	82,079	83,505	-1,426	-2%
Interest Expense	2,315	2,044	271	13%
Laundry	375	378	-3	-1%
Licenses and Permits	1,931	158	1,773	1122%
Loan Expense	0	49,772	-49,772	-100%
Medical	3,022	2,291	731	32%
Medical Supplies	1,859	1,012	847	84%
Mortgage	13,718	13,719	-1	0%
Office	16,454	68,217	-51,763	-76%
Payroll	93,427	92,247	1,180	1%
Pension Management	5,734	2,801	2,933	105%
Petty Cash	743	743	0	0%
Postage & Delivery	3,664	1,766	1,898	107%
Professional Development	6,758	5,989	769	13%
Professional Fees	10,597	13,212	-2,615	-20%
Refunds	107,481	60,590	46,891	77%
Subscriptions	555	850	-295	-35%
Tax	27,759	990	26,769	2704%
Telephone	15,873	11,733	4,140	35%
Trash Removal	745	615	130	21%
Travel & Entertainment	198	245	-47	-19%
Uncategorized Expenses	0	0	0	0%
Utilities	2,440	1,895	545	29%
Total Expense	446,676	459,255	-12,579	-3%
Net Income	681,907	705,534	-23,627	-3%

This kind of report can be extremely useful to you, not only in understanding the period in question, but also in relating that time period to a comparable time, such as the previous quarter or the same quarter of the prior year. Both revenues and costs can be arranged side-by-side and the variance calculated either in dollar amount or percentage amount (see same figure). Examining these variances can point you in a new direction to explore problems or opportunities.

Costs

Clearly, financial statements don't tell the entire story. The nature of a medical practice, like any business, is as an ongoing, ever-changing, almost living, breathing beast! Most physicians are not exposed at any point in their training to cost management, and yet, it affects us greatly on a daily basis. In fact, in my experience, those of us who have any "business" education or direction from our senior partners, our chairmen, or our administrators are directed, almost exclusively, to focus on the revenue side of the equation.

We are taught how to code correctly for procedures that we perform, so as to maximize reimbursements. We are told which insurance companies to "accept" so that we can build our practice with patients who have those plans.

Our exposure to understanding and managing costs is typically very limited. We're told that we can go only to this conference or that one...for how many days we can attend...and how many medical societies we can join if we would like for our membership dues to be covered by our practice or department. The only explanation we're given is "cost."

It is uncommon for physicians, even in private practice, to pay a great deal of attention to the cost side of practicing medicine. This is an enormous mistake that has profound implications for both your practice profitability and your income.

By understanding the nature of costs and their behavior, you can more effectively evaluate how to manage them to maximize the profitability of your medical practice.

For our purposes, the best way to classify cost behavior is in two categories. The first is called "fixed" costs and the second is "variable" costs. Let's look at each of them and review examples of both.

A fixed cost is one that does not change, regardless of the activity of the business or practice. Whether you see one patient or a hundred in any given time period, whether you take a vacation or not, whether your patients are Medicaid or self-pay, fixed costs remain the same. This kind of behavior is represented graphically in Figure 3.4:

Figure 3.4: Fixed Costs

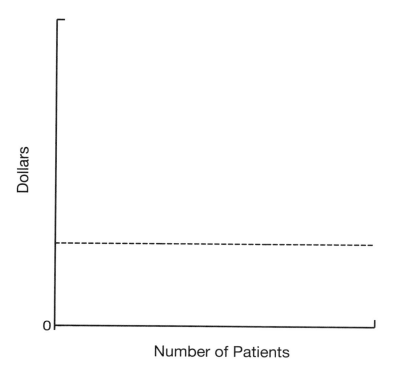

Examples of typical fixed costs in a medical practice are rent, salaries, malpractice insurance, and debt service on capital equipment.

Variable costs, in contrast, change according to the level of activity of a practice. The more patients you see, or the more times you do a procedure, or the more days that you are in the office, the more variable costs are incurred. This is graphically represented in Figure 3.5.

Figure 3.5: Variable Costs

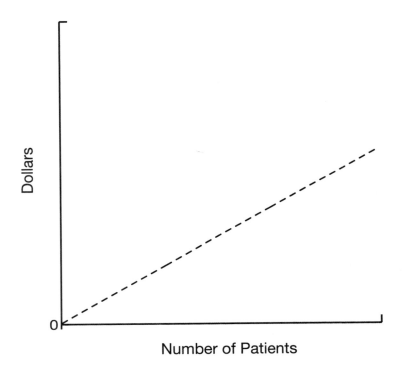

Examples of variable costs in a medical practice are disposables (things like sponges and syringes), non-capital equipment, utilities, overtime pay, and other productivity bonuses. Variable costs are those costs that are incurred incrementally with each use.

Essentially, you can consider that fixed costs, in aggregate, for a medical practice, are those costs that allow you to open your doors. Variable costs are those which are additive in your ability to take care of patients. Combined, they make up the total costs of the practice.

Figure 3.6: Total Costs

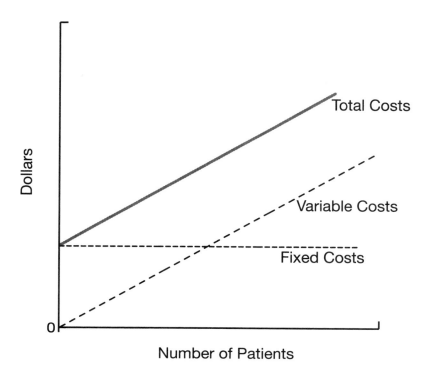

Understanding these relationships is imperative to maintaining the viability of a medical practice, or for that matter, any business entity.

Putting It All Together

Let's build a graphical model to better understand the relationship between costs, volumes, and revenues, so that we can better manage them.

Figure 3.7 shows a blank graph where the x-axis represents the number of patients seen on an annual basis in a medical practice, and the y-axis represents dollars.

Figure 3.7: Revenue and Patient Volume

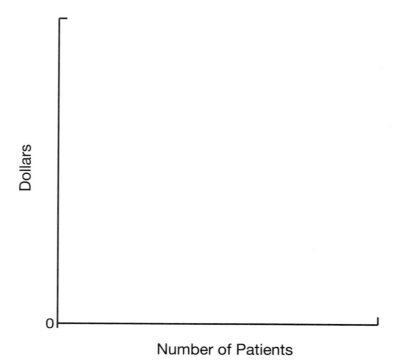

In the next figure, I've added a dashed line representing fixed costs. As you can see, this is a horizontal line, because, as explained previously, fixed costs do not change regardless of the number of patients seen.

Figure 3.8: Cost Behavior: Fixed Costs

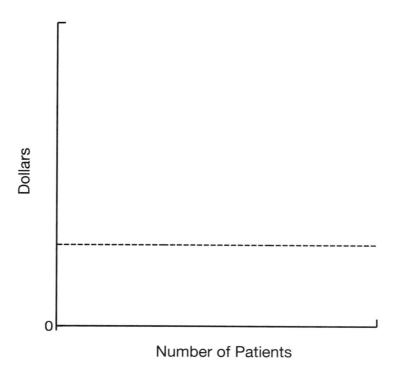

You should know that the point at which this line intersects the y-axis is the cost of opening your doors before even a single patient has been seen.

The line in the next figure represents variable costs. For the sake of simplicity, I've made this a straight line. In the real world, you can imagine that, for a variety of reasons, the variable costs line will often change, depending on a variety of situations.

Figure 3.9: Cost Behavior: Variable Costs

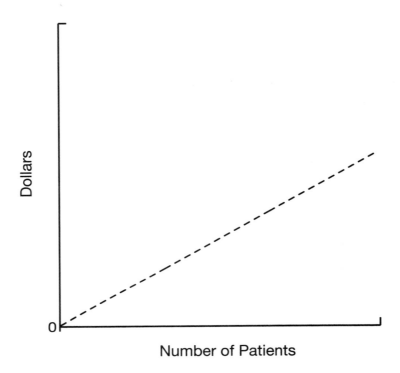

For example, you can imagine that if you buy sponges in bulk, your cost basis will change as you buy more. This is a built-in incentive, from the vendor, to get you to purchase more of his product. So, for a single variable cost like sponges, the graph may look more like the next figure.

Figure 3.10: A More Accurate Variable Costs Curve

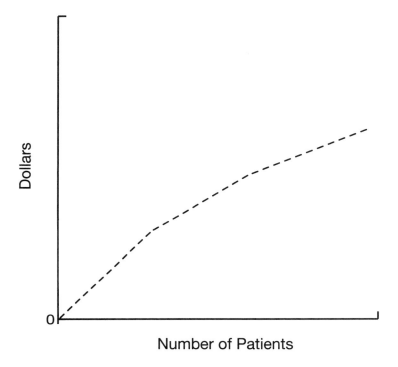

Back to our larger model. In the next figure, I have added a gray line, which represents total costs (the sum of fixed and variable costs). As you can see, the total costs increase as more patients are seen.

Figure 3.11: Total Costs

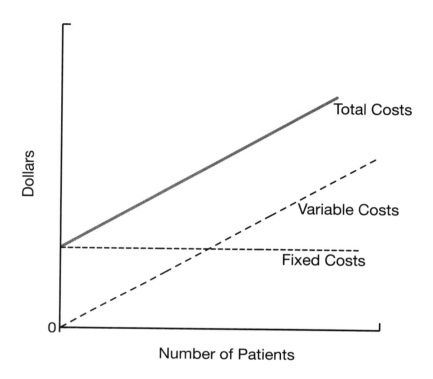

The black line in the next figure represents revenues, or total sales. Again, for simplicity's sake, I am assuming equivalent revenue from each additional patient seen. Of course, this is grossly oversimplified, but will serve for our purposes here.

Figure 3.12: Total Revenues

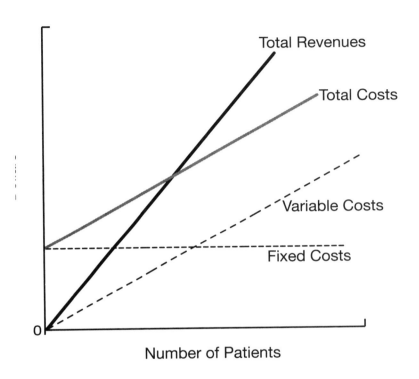

The point at which total revenues equals total costs is known as the break-even point. (See Figure 3.13.)

Figure 3.13: Break-even Point

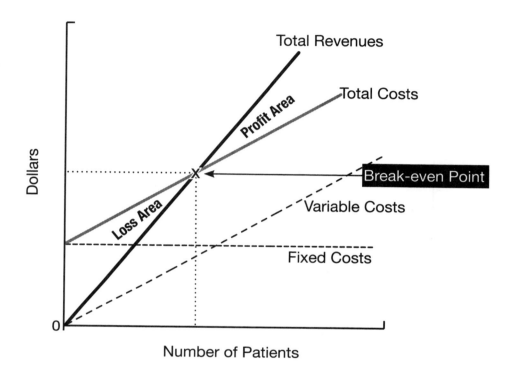

A vertical line down from that point shows how many patients need to be seen in order to break even. Any additional patient seen generates profit, whereas, the practice incurs a loss if it sees fewer patients. The triangle created in the upper right of the graph is the profit area; the triangle in the lower left is known as the loss area.

So what happens if we change some of these variables? First, let's look at the graph if we lower our fixed costs.

Figure 3.14: Understanding Cost Behavior: Reducing Fixed Costs

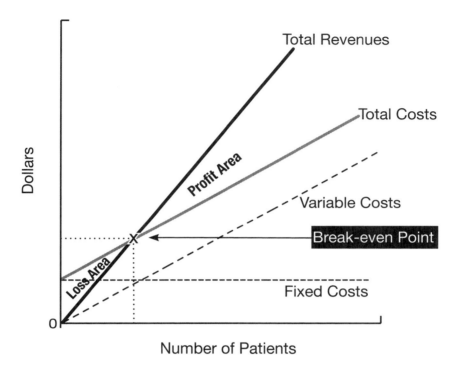

Clearly, the break-even point shifts to the left and fewer patients need to be seen to begin to earn profit. However, the slope of the line does not change, and the profitability of each incremental patient does not increase.

On the other hand, if we were to reduce the variable costs rather than the fixed costs (see Figure 3.15), the break-even point does not shift as much, but the profit area improves dramatically. That area represents the magnitude of the profit at a given point on the x-axis. More separation of the lines that show total costs and total revenues means more profit.

Figure 3.15: Understanding Cost Behavior: Reducing Variable Costs

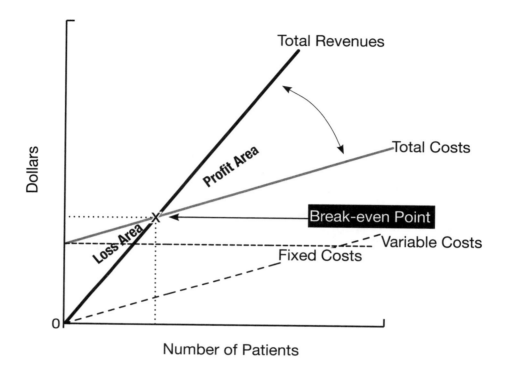

In the case where variable costs are low, each additional patient or procedure produces more incremental profit. We will come back to this concept in Chapter 4, in the section on "Contribution Margin."

In order to understand this better, let's look again at the simple graph on the behavior of fixed costs. Remember Figure 3.4 from earlier in this chapter? On Figure 3.16, I have superimposed a line representing cost per patient of this same fixed cost.

Figure 3.16: Understanding Cost Behavior: Fixed Costs

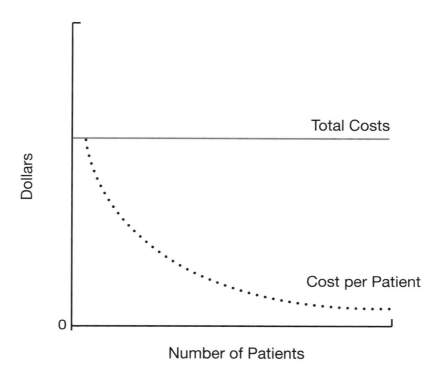

As you can see, the cost per patient diminishes rapidly with each use of a fixed cost, and the curve ultimately smoothes. Either way, with each use of a piece of equipment, office, or whatever the fixed cost represents, your cost per patient is lower.

On the other hand, the next figure shows the cost per patient of a variable cost. It is the same for each use.

Figure 3.17: Understand Cost Behavior: Variable Costs

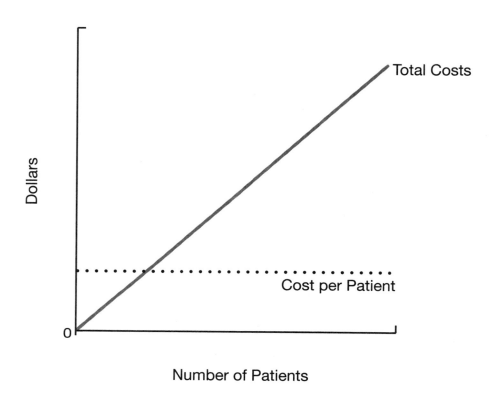

Remember that variable costs don't necessarily act in a straight line. But for these types of costs, we spend money each time we perform a service.

It should be apparent, then, that for low volume events, it pays to keep fixed costs as low as possible and shift whatever costs possible into the variable cost behavior pattern.

For example: Suppose you perform a certain type of minor procedure approximately once a month. You could buy a machine costing $80,000 and use it as often as you need. Or, you could rent the use of someone else's machine for $50 per patient. You would have to do 1,600 of these procedures to justify the "fixed" cost of buying the machine. That would take more than 130 years! In this example, since your break-even point is unattainable, it is clearly better to rent the machine rather than to buy one.

The exact opposite is true for high-volume events. For these, it is best to keep variable costs low. We will discuss this further in the following chapter, "So, You Want to Buy a New Toy?" Read on to learn how to use these financial tools to choose among opportunities that compete for resources and to anticipate and adjust for actual practice performance.

Key Learning Points: Numbers You SHOULD Know (Everyone Else Does)

1. Understand cash basis versus accrual basis accounting, the chart of accounts, assets and liabilities, basic financial statements, and the nature of costs and revenues.

2. Learn how to manage fixed and variable costs for the profitability of your practice and your income.

3. Understand the relationship between cost, volume, and profit by plotting the break-even point for the number of patients your practice needs to see.

4. For low volume events, it pays to keep fixed costs as low as possible and shift costs into the variable cost pattern. For high volume events, the reverse is true.

CHAPTER 4
SO, YOU WANT TO BUY A NEW TOY?

· · · · · · · · · · ·

Not too long ago, I served as the director of business development for my Department of Surgery. Within a very brief period of time, I was approached by four of my colleagues about projects of interest to them.

The first was a young colleague who felt that we should purchase a laser in order to perform laser vein ablation for her patients with lower extremity venous disease. The second wanted an ultrasound machine, for use in his office, in order to evaluate head and neck lesions. A division chief approached me about the possibility of bringing on a young recruit, and a friend and colleague in private practice asked me to help him decide whether or not he should perform gastric banding for patients with morbid obesity.

All four, while proposing different programs, sounded remarkably similar in their approach:

"It's really cool. It would be such a great thing."
"The patients will absolutely love it. They're asking for it all the time."
"They're doing it up the street at Columbia."
"It's not that expensive, and we could make a lot of money."

Tell me if this sounds familiar to you. I am certain that virtually every one of you reading this has made or heard a similar argument.

The problem is that the people who hold the purse strings, and who are in a position to provide the resources for such new endeavors, evaluate these programs in a language much different from this. In this chapter, we will build upon the concepts outlined in Chapters 2 and 3 to learn how to critically evaluate new programs and technologies (including service lines, capital equipment, and physician recruits) and to present these analyses in the manner and format required by the decision makers in your organization.

By presenting proposals using business plans—and by evaluating contribution margins and performing break-even analysis, target analysis, and anticipated return on investment—for a new program or a technology, you will maximize your ability to secure and utilize the resources of your institution in order to promote new methods of treatment for your patients.

It is critical to understand, at the outset, that these analyses don't have to be "right" in order to be effective. In fact, they are never "right." The difference is that by presenting your proposals in this manner, the suits who hold the financial purse strings are much more open to continuing the discussion with you, rather than merely shutting you down and saying no. This kind of dialogue goes a long way toward creating a true partnership between physicians and administration, which is a hallmark of all successful healthcare organizations of any size.

By demonstrating that you have given thought to return on investment, for example, you improve your credibility. You demonstrate that your goals align with those of the organization. As a result, financial decision makers will look forward to working with you to negotiate a workable plan. So, in preparing for the negotiation, make an effort to put some numbers into your proposal, but also recognize the numbers will virtually always change. Let's explore some key terms you'll need to know to be successful.

Business Plans

The term "business plan" is a widely used phrase that can refer to any of a variety of documents meant to outline a financial proposal. This can range from a simple scribble on the back of a cocktail napkin to a formal, bound, multi-chapter strategic plan for an organization. Fortunately, for our purposes, we can lean more toward the simpler forms.

In most medical settings, a business plan can take the form of a relatively simple spreadsheet that contains one or several model scenarios for a proposed project. Let's use the recruitment of a new physician as a model. Figure 4.1 is an example of a five-year business plan for a young physician right out of training.

Figure 4.1: Example Five-Year Business Plan

Christina Yang, MD	Year 1 Projected	Year 2 Projected	Year 3 Projected	Year 4 Projected	Year 5 Projected
REVENUE					
Estimated Gross Receipts	$150,000	$225,000	$275,000	$450,000	$500,000
Research Grant Support	-	-	-	-	-
Other Support	$100,000	$100,000	$100,000	-	-
Total Revenue	$250,000	$325,000	$375,000	$450,000	$500,000
EXPENSES					
Compensation Model	Guaranteed Salary	Guaranteed Salary	Guaranteed Salary	Productivity Model	Productivity Model
MD Salary	$90,000	$90,000	$90,000	$90,000	$90,000
MD Fringe Benefits	$24,750	$24,750	$24,750	$24,750	$24,750
Guaranteed Supplement	$110,000	$110,000	$110,000	-	-
Productivity Supplement	-	-	-	$135,000	$160,000
Staff Salaries (5% increase per year)	$45,000	$47,250	$49,613	$52,093	$54,698
Staff Fringe	$12,375	$12,994	$13,643	$14,326	$15,042
Subtotal	$282,125	$284,994	$288,006	$316,169	$344,490
Practice OTPS (5% increase per year)	$5,000	$5,250	$5,513	$5,788	$6,078
Rent	$5,000	$5,250	$5,513	$5,788	$6,078
Malpractice Insurance	$25,000	$26,250	$27,563	$28,941	$30,388
Subtotal	$30,000	$31,500	$33,075	$34,729	$36,465
Taxes					
School Taxes 11.4%	$17,100	$25,650	$31,350	$51,300	$57,000
Department Tax 10%	$15,000	$22,500	$27,500	$45,000	$50,000
Subtotal Taxes	$32,100	$48,150	$58,850	$96,300	$107,000
TOTAL EXPENSES	$349,225	$369,894	$385,443	$452,986	$494,032
Reinvestment of Department Tax	$15,000	$22,500	$27,500	-	-
SURPLUS/(DEFICIT)	**$(84,225)**	**$(22,394)**	**$17,057**	**$(2,986)**	**$5,968**

At first blush, this looks like a highly detailed and accurate assessment of the cost and profitability (or lack thereof) of this new, young doctor. Don't let the numbers scare you or fool you.

When you look closely, many of the fields contain numbers that come from the standards of the business in question. For example, MD and staff salaries are fixed costs that can be determined at the outset (at least for the first three years of the model). These are simply plugged into the spreadsheet. Below the MD salary and the staff salaries are lines for "fringe benefits."

Most organizations have a fixed fringe benefit calculation that allows for this number to be derived from the number immediately above it. In this case, the fringe benefits are calculated by multiplying both the physician and staff salaries by 27.5 percent. Other fixed costs, such as malpractice insurance, are also easily populated into the business plan.

As an aside, I have utilized an accounting tool that you should recognize, either as an employee or as a manager. You will note that the MD compensation has three components to it: MD salary, MD fringe benefits, and either "guaranteed supplement" in the first three years, or "productivity supplement" in the final two years.

In this scenario, my friend the division chief has promised the new doctor a "guarantee" of $200,000 for each of the first three years. This consists of a salary of $90,000 and a guaranteed supplement of $110,000. You will notice that the fringe benefits are based only on the salary piece, saving the practice or department 27.5 percent of the other $110,000, or $30,250 in each of the first three years!

	Guaranteed Salary	Guaranteed Salary	Guaranteed Salary	Guaranteed Salary	Guaranteed Salary
MD Salary	$90,000	$90,000	$90,000	$90,000	$90,000
MD Fringe Benefits	$24,750	$24,750	$24,750	$24,750	$24,750
Guaranteed Supplement	$110,000	$110,000	$110,000	-	-
Productivity Supplement	-	-	-	$135,000	$160,000

In the fourth and fifth years of our model, the physician has been placed on a productivity model, in which her combined salary and productivity supplement are equal to 50 percent of her total revenue. The savings to the department on the fringe benefits of the projected supplements are even greater in these two years.

Other elements of this example are worth noting. In this scenario, we have built in three years of external support for $100,000 a year. You can see that, even with this kind of support, the bottom line is still negative (a loss) to the department. The department (and the external supporter, often either a hospital or medical school) is making a significant investment, which begins to pay back only in year three.

You also see what is a fairly typical tax structure in a large academic institution in which the dean (the school) and the department tax receipts at a fixed rate. It costs a lot to run a medical school! Our department here has reinvested its tax in the first three years to further support the new recruit.

"OTPS" is a standard accounting acronym for "Other Than Personal Services." These are essentially the supplies and "stuff" that someone will use over the course of the year, and can be either a "guesstimate" or an actual accounting. But these, as you shall soon see, are "nickels and dimes."

You'll note, at the top, that the first row of numbers contains estimated gross receipts. Here is where the plan gets really fuzzy. Many people call this kind of business plan a "blue sky analysis," because the numbers that are used to formulate the proposal are plucked out of the clear, blue sky. This top line is an example of such an analysis.

Where do these numbers come from? The person creating the plan, if he or she is smart, will try to base this estimation on as many data points as possible. For example, is there a history of the receipts of a new physician coming in at this level? What does the market look like? Does this physician have a particular skill set that is missing from the practice that she is going to bring to the table? Is she replacing another practitioner? What is the payer mix of the expected population of patients?

At the end of the day, this number is still an estimate and still, to some degree, blue sky, but every attempt is made to be as critical as possible in creating these assumptions. Figure 4.2 shows the outcome if these assumptions prove to be incorrect.

Figure 4.2: Five-Year Business Plan: Actual Performance

Christina Yang, MD	Year 1 Actual	Year 2 Actual	Year 3 Actual	Year 4 Actual	Year 5 Actual
REVENUE					
Gross Receipts	$97,487	$169,814	$227,642	$279,391	$346,221
Research Grant Support	-	-	-	-	-
Other Support	$100,000	$100,000	$100,000	-	-
Total Revenue	$197,487	$269,814	$327,642	$279,391	$346,221
EXPENSES					
Compensation Model	Guaranteed Salary	Guaranteed Salary	Guaranteed Salary	**Productivity Model**	**Productivity Model**
MD Salary	$90,000	$90,000	$90,000	$90,000	$90,000
MD Fringe Benefits	$24,750	$24,750	$24,750	$24,750	$24,750
Guaranteed Supplement	$110,000	$110,000	$110,000	-	-
Productivity Supplement	-	-	-	$49,696	$83,111
Staff Salaries (5% increase per year)	$45,000	$47,250	$49,613	$52,093	$54,698
Staff Fringe	$12,375	$12,994	$13,643	$14,326	$15,042
Subtotal	$282,125	$284,994	$288,006	$230,864	$267,600
Practice OTPS (5% increase per year)	$5,000	$5,250	$5,513	$5,788	$6,078
Rent	$5,000	$5,250	$5,513	$5,788	$6,078
Malpractice Insurance	$25,000	$26,250	$27,563	$28,941	$30,388
Subtotal	$30,000	$31,500	$33,075	$34,729	$36,465
Taxes					
School Taxes 11.4%	$11,114	$19,359	$25,951	$31,851	$39,469
Department Tax 10%	$9,749	$16,981	$22,764	$27,939	$34,622
Subtotal Taxes	$20,862	$36,340	$48,715	$59,790	$74,091
TOTAL EXPENSES	$337,987	$358,084	$375,309	$331,171	$384,234
Reinvestment of Department Tax	$9,749	$16,981	$22,764	-	-
SURPLUS/(DEFICIT)	$(130,752)	$(71,289)	$(24,903)	$(51,780)	$(38,013)

When our young recruit fails to bring in the kind of revenues we projected, everybody loses. The department's loss over the five-year period shown is almost a quarter of a million dollars more than projected, and the physician herself actually takes home significantly less in years four ($139, 696) and five ($173,111) than in years one through three ($200,000).

In any event, the creation of a document such as this encourages both the physician and you to realistically examine the financial implications of your proposed new hire. When creating a business plan like this, it is helpful to use a spreadsheet program and to "play with" the numbers in a variety of different ways.

Create "best," "middle," and "worst" case projections by changing the revenue numbers. See what happens if the hospital were to reduce its support in Year 2. What if space costs increase? What if the dean changes the tax structure? Any of these scenarios can be plugged into the model, and the bottom line immediately changes to reflect the new reality.

This is also a useful tool for tracking performance as you follow your new, young associate's progress through the five years of the model. Hopefully, by performing a regular review of this exercise, you will avoid the disaster that has befallen our division chief in the example above.

Contribution Margin

Hospitals love contribution margin. Try this experiment. Go to the chief operating officer of your hospital and ask him what the five top procedures are in the hospital, with respect to contribution margin. I guarantee you his eyes will light up and he will talk so fast that you may be unable to follow him. It is simply because this metric is so important to hospital operations that you must understand it and know where you fit in, from a hospital's point of view. Additionally, this concept will be invaluable in evaluating new technologies for your own practice.

Simply put, contribution margin is the amount of money that each additional procedure or patient adds to the bottom line. Formulaically, contribution margin equals incremental revenue (the additional money received for each procedure or patient) minus variable costs.

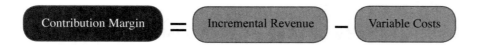

Contribution Margin = Incremental Revenue − Variable Costs

As we saw earlier, variable costs are not the only costs that go into a procedure or program. However, because your fixed costs don't change, regardless of how many patients you see or procedures you do, this metric ignores those fixed costs and tells you how much additional money you will have in your pocket from the next patient or procedure. Once fixed costs have been covered, contribution margin is pure profit.

For example, let's say that the laser vein procedure, proposed earlier, will provide $100 of additional revenue each time it is performed. (A more sophisticated analysis will take into account your payer mix and the varying reimbursements expected from each payer. You can use these to formulate the average expected revenue. In this case, we are using $100 for ease of illustration.) The clinical supplies required (variable costs) are a laser catheter and some sponges and syringes. Let's assume that these add up to $20. The contribution margin for this procedure is:

$$\underset{\text{(Contribution Margin)}}{\$80.00} = \underset{\text{(Incremental Revenue)}}{\$100.00} - \underset{\text{(Variable Costs)}}{\$20.00}$$

Therefore, each time you do a laser vein procedure, you are bringing $80 of additional profit into the practice.

Sounds like a no-brainer, right? Not so fast, though. We still haven't taken into account the cost of the machine itself (fixed cost). So contribution margin, alone, is not enough to evaluate the wisdom or feasibility of a project or technology. For a more complete picture, we need to perform a break-even analysis.

Break-even Analysis

A break-even analysis takes into account both fixed and variable costs in calculating the true financial value of a procedure or piece of equipment. It is a way to calculate the number of times a procedure must be performed, or the number of patients who must be seen, in order to, well, break even. Formulaically, the break-even point, in number of procedures, equals fixed cost divided by contribution margin.

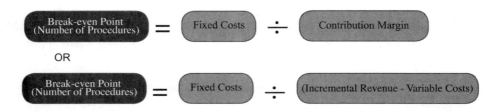

If the machine in question, our laser vein machine, costs $80,000, then the break-even point equals $80,000 divided by the contribution margin of $80 per case, for a result of 1,000 cases.

This tells us that in order to break even, our vascular surgeon needs to do 1,000 procedures just to pay for the machine. Our contribution margin equation tells us that the 1,001st patient will yield us $80 of pure profit.

In determining whether or not to embark on such an endeavor, this is the starting point at which you can decide whether this machine is worth it. Back to our blue sky analysis. We need to determine, as best we can, whether or not this physician is likely to perform 1,000 procedures, and over what period of time.

Target Analysis

Target analysis is a variant of break-even analysis that builds in proposed additional revenue for working capital, loan repayment, or (oh, yes!) physician compensation. Using our previous example, if we determined that in order to make a laser vein program worth our while, we would require a $16,000 profit, our target analysis would incorporate that in the numerator of the break-even analysis, along with the fixed costs. Our new break-even point, or target point, is equal to fixed costs plus the target. That sum is then divided by the contribution margin to tell us how many procedures we need to perform.

Target Point (# of Procedures Needed) = (Fixed Costs + Targeted Profit) ÷ Contribution Margin

In this case, our target point equals $80,000 (the fixed cost) plus our target of $16,000 to equal $96,000. This sum, divided by our $80 contribution margin, yields a result of 1,200 procedures that would need to be performed in order to make this "worthwhile" in our minds.

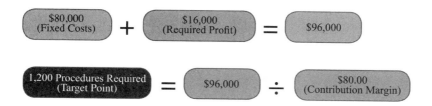

$80,000 (Fixed Costs) + $16,000 (Required Profit) = $96,000

1,200 Procedures Required (Target Point) = $96,000 ÷ $80.00 (Contribution Margin)

These kinds of analyses are simple and quick and will go a long way toward having your proposal taken seriously by your partners in administration.

Return on Investment

Return on investment (ROI) conversations can be very tricky, in large part because there are as many formulae to calculate ROI as there are investments on which to calculate the returns. Essentially, from a straight accounting point of view, ROI is the gain, usually expressed as a percentage, from having spent money on an investment or project. Formulaically, ROI can be expressed as follows:

$$\boxed{ROI} = \boxed{(Net\ Revenue - Costs)} \div \boxed{Costs}$$

In our laser vein project above, if we meet our target of 1,200 cases (we are not factoring time in our analysis here), we can expect a rate of return of 20 percent.

$$\boxed{\substack{20\ \% \\ (ROI)}} = \boxed{\substack{\$96,000 - \$80,000 \\ (Net\ Revenue - Costs)}} \div \boxed{\substack{\$80,000 \\ (Costs)}}$$

Note: For simplicity, I am excluding the variable cost of $20 per procedure from both the revenue side and the cost side of this equation.

In a sophisticated financial environment, ROI is often used to compare the relative values of competing potential investments. Assume, for a moment, that you are managing a small group practice, and the vascular surgeon in your group just came to you with her laser vein proposal. Moments later, the head and neck surgeon approaches you about the office ultrasound machine. Let's say, for example, that a new ultrasound machine costs $50,000. You perform a careful analysis using the tools outlined above, which shows that over a four-year period, you can anticipate a net revenue of $62,000, or a profit of $12,000, if you buy the new machine.

You are a wise senior partner, and you recognize the need to make sizable investments in the growth of your practice. But you're not awash in cash, and you can approve only one of these projects. At first blush, it might seem that the $16,000 profit from the laser would be more beneficial than the $12,000 from the ultrasound. Or maybe it would be better to spend only $50,000 on the ultrasound rather than $80,000 on the laser.

The ROI calculation takes both considerations into account. You calculate that the ROI of the ultrasound is 24 percent:

$$\underset{\text{(ROI)}}{24\,\%} = \underset{\text{(Net Revenue - Costs)}}{\$62{,}000 - \$50{,}000} \div \underset{\text{(Costs)}}{\$50{,}000}$$

The return on your investment in the ultrasound is higher (24 percent) than that of the laser (20 percent); so, using this method of calculation, the ultrasound may be a "better" use of capital.

Another Way of Thinking about ROI

I want to caution you here about overusing the tools we have reviewed in this chapter and in this entire section of the book. Absolutely, you need to be familiar with their use and be conversant with these terms. This will make you an excellent partner in the back office of your practice, in your department administrator's meetings, and in the boardroom of your hospital or health system. These concepts are critical for you to survive and thrive as a physician in any size practice in these challenging times, whether you are a partner or an employee. Do not forget that.

But to rely exclusively on financial analysis to make all of your practice decisions ignores your prime motivation: to provide outstanding care to your patients and their families... to feel a sense of purpose, worthwhile work, and making a difference.

Remember my friend who was deciding whether he should add bariatric surgery to his practice? We did the financial analysis together, first on the back of a napkin and then on a spreadsheet. What we found was that, financially, it was essentially a wash. He would make money, but not necessarily enough to justify the investment in new equipment, office furniture, special exam tables, etc. That is, the calculated ROI was fairly low.

And yet, he chose to do it anyway. He felt that he was able to connect with these patients in a way that was intrinsically satisfying to him, and the visible result of the surgeries was a source of real pride for him.

And his practice exploded. Not only did he develop a large bariatric surgical practice, but his general surgical practice took off as well. Why? He became increasingly well-regarded in his community as a doctor who delivered exceptional care to his patients. These days, he and I are discussing blue sky projections for adding a potential junior partner to his practice. How's that for ROI?

A Word about Employees

In your practice, your most important asset is your staff. And, while your employees may show up in your P&L as costs, the successful physician views the people around him or her as investments.

What do employees want in a leader like you? They want approachability, tools and equipment to do their jobs well, appreciation, efficient systems, and opportunities for professional development. Remember, when you give employees the resources and information they need to effectively serve you and your patients, you'll earn an impressive ROI through greater patient loyalty and higher market share. Ultimately, your practice will enjoy a reputation for excellence, and you will turn a profit.

Key Learning Points: So, You Want to Buy a New Toy?

1. While purchasing a new ultrasound machine, recruiting a new specialist, or offering patients a new surgical procedure would, of course, be really cool, you are more likely to actually get your proposal funded by developing and presenting a business plan.

2. Many of the numbers and data you will need to populate a simple spreadsheet are standard business formulas that are readily available.

3. Don't expect your analysis to be "right." The numbers will change. You should view the exercise as a starting point for a conversation.

4. Contribution margin, break-even analysis, target analysis, and ROI are fairly simple calculations that may be used to provide an educated guess as to the profitability of a proposed program.

5. ROI is ultimately about more than money. Give high consideration to decisions that positively impact your employees, patients, and your personal job satisfaction.

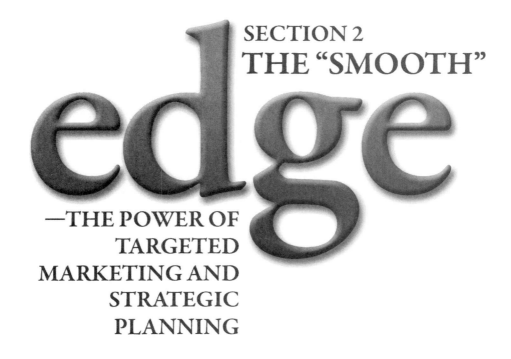

SECTION 2
THE "SMOOTH"
edge
—THE POWER OF TARGETED MARKETING AND STRATEGIC PLANNING

Your ability to understand your medical practice's position in the market, to protect and grow market share, and to plan for the future is more critical than ever.

Consider this email that I recently received from a leader of a large radiology practice. He wrote:

> My managers and I would like to come by sometime to meet with you and your team to discuss ways we can provide imaging services to your patients. We can offer block time, if you wish, and work it around your office hours, if that is of interest. Please let us know when it would be convenient for you and your team.

This is a potentially highly effective move that underscores the importance of this section. We will come back to this story later to review the genius (and failure) of this particular note. But it demonstrates that the techniques, tools, and "numbers" that we reviewed in the previous section will mean little (and be little) without understanding the critical value of marketing and strategic planning.

CHAPTER 5

MARKETING IS *NOT* ADVERTISING
· · · · · · · · · ·

Marketing is not advertising, although advertising is part of marketing. Ask any doctor, or for that matter almost anybody, about marketing, and I guarantee you he will respond with something like this:

Marketing is great. If only we had the money to do newspaper ads and TV ads, it would really be helpful to our business.
We need a logo.
We need a slogan.

While all of these are potentially part of a business's or medical practice's overall marketing strategy, they represent but a small part of what is truly important in marketing and strategic planning. Those who live in the New York area surely remember riding the subway in the late '70s and early '80s and seeing the sign for "laser hemorrhoids."

This was one of the first blatant advertising ploys from a physician practice. Prior to this, and even then, it was considered lowbrow to advertise a medical practice. And really, how many people do you suppose wrote down that number and called 1-800-MD-TUSHY to have that physician perform surgery on such a delicate part of the anatomy? Nobody I know.

True—and effective—marketing is much bigger than that. Marketing and strategic planning include the idea of determining who and what you are, what image you want to project, whom you service, and how to provide your customer base with what they need. Remember the advice of my senior partner when I initially joined the practice? He said, "Remember the three A's of success: Be Affable, Able, and Available." And again, the focus was on availability. He may not have realized it, but this really was a fairly complete and successful marketing strategy.

Ability, as we shall discuss again, is really the price of entry in medicine today. We all like to think that we are better than our competitors. However, in planning for our own success, we have to allow for the reality that our competitors are pretty good, too.

So that leaves availability and affability. Here is where we can differentiate ourselves from our competition. It is this ability to demonstrate how we are unique that allows us to capture market share from our competition. In my case, 17 years ago, and even more so for you now, given the constraints on your practice, affability and availability have real potential to be differentiating characteristics.

The Five Ps of Marketing

Marketing professionals will often talk about the "Five Ps" of marketing. They are:
- Product
- Price
- Place
- Promotion
- Positioning

In its simplest form, "product" is the good (or service) that you are offering to your customers. Whatever your medical specialty, you have a service offering that has some distinguishing characteristics from that of other doctors or practices. At the very least, your offering is distinct from that of those in other specialties.

But do you have any unique services that may differentiate you from your real competition? For example: Are you an early adopter of a new technology? Do you have a shorter length of stay for a particular procedure? Do you have a nutritionist as part of your practice? This is something that is worth exploring in your own practice.

"Price" is interesting when it comes to medical services. Certainly, there was a time when one could expect to make deals with patients, or people who controlled patient purchasing behaviors, in order to gain volume and market share. The quintessential example of this was in the mid- to late-1980s when HMOs came on the scene. Prior to this, price was really a non-issue.

One of the reasons the HMOs were able to expand so rapidly throughout healthcare was their ability to instill fear into physicians...fear that they would lose their patient base if they would not more aggressively price their services. Tens of thousands of doctors joined HMOs as a result.

What we are seeing now, with declining reimbursement across the board, is a direct result of our reaction to this phenomenon. In many respects, we have become a "commodity," defined by Webster as "a good or service whose wide availability typically leads to smaller profit margins and diminishes the importance of factors (such as brand name) other than price."

In a sense, the market has tried to render us physicians interchangeable. Currently, price is not a particularly useful marketing strategy for physicians, with certain exceptions. If you perform a purely cosmetic procedure, for example, you might be able to create package pricing deals that are attractive to your patient base. For the most part, other specialties are no longer in a position to engage in a price war.

"Place" refers to your distribution channel. It refers to where, and in which environments, you offer your services. In the outpatient setting, this can mean the small community practice versus the large inner-city clinic. On the inpatient side, it has to do with the hospital or medical center with which you are affiliated. Place can have important implications and a huge effect on the nature of your patient base and your ability to grow and protect your market share.

"Promotion" refers to your ability to raise awareness with your target market. This is where advertising begins to come into the mix. But in addition to that, your relationships with a variety of different groups of people, including your referring physicians, the leadership of your medical center, and your community, can have a great deal of impact on the growth of your practice.

"Positioning" refers to how your market defines you in relation to your competition. This is not the physical space or place that we discussed earlier, but can be thought of as the place that your name holds in the minds of your target groups. For example, although I am a general surgeon by training, in the minds of my market, I am the Crohn's and Colitis guy. Nobody would think to send me a thyroid patient. This is where your ability to create a point of differentiation from your competition is so critical.

In medicine, it is the last two Ps, promotion and positioning, on which you should focus in order to create a strategic plan to grow and protect your patient base.

The remainder of the chapter will focus mainly on these points.

Try This Experiment

Next time you're in a room with 20 or more doctors, ask the following question: Why should I go to you rather than the guy sitting next to you? What makes you different from the woman in front of you? What, in marketing-speak, is your "point of differentiation"? I have seen this experiment performed several times, and the outcome has always been the same. In fact, I am certain that right now, as you are thinking to yourself, *How would I answer that question?* one word comes to mind: quality.

Each of the first five people you ask will use that word: quality. By about the sixth person or so, everyone will see the fault in this line of reasoning and alter their responses. It is then that you will start to see what is truly a potential point of differentiation: service. Even there, though, people are reluctant to believe that the service they provide is inferior to that of their competition.

Ask a room full of doctors to raise their hands if any of them think that they are below average in terms of quality. You will not see a single hand. Any hand you see should not be in this line of work. Ask again who provides inferior service, and again, not a single hand will go up. Can this be accurate?

Don't misunderstand me. I do not mean to diminish the importance and value of quality in healthcare. Quite the opposite. In our profession, the stakes are so high that anything short of the highest quality of care is completely unacceptable. Quality is the price of entry, the bare minimum, and every patient, physician, and healthcare facility should demand it. Only after we achieve this can we begin to address how we differentiate ourselves from our competitors.

Public Reporting of Quality

I am concerned that our profession's limited ability to measure comparative quality data—and our patients' limited ability to interpret them—may lead people to make erroneous conclusions about individual institutions and/or physicians.

Can the quality of a medical practice be measured in an objective way? A renewed national focus on quality has the potential, in the next few years, to actually be a measurable point of differentiation. This can be good or, more likely, very bad for many of us. If you haven't yet visited the Center for Medicare and Medicaid Service's (CMS) website, hospitalcompare.hhs.gov, then you are woefully behind the curve.

I suggest you put this book down now, log on, and see how your hospital stacks up against local competitors on very specific quality indicators. Increasingly, this is where consumers will go before they choose a hospital. I guarantee you that many of your patients have seen this site. If they haven't, they soon will, as the CMS has taken out full-page ads in every major urban newspaper in the country to promote its existence.

And if you ever thought that patient satisfaction was "soft stuff," it's time to revise your opinion. HCAHPS—or Hospital Consumer Assessment of Healthcare Providers and Systems—is a CMS standardized quality initiative that measures patients' perception of care.

It surveys adult inpatients on a frequency scale. In other words, the web-site reports "top box" scores (the percentage of patients who reported hospital staff, nurses, or physicians "always" did a behavior versus, say, sometimes or never) for each hospital on six categories of questions that include things like communication with doctors, communication about medications, and pain management, to name a few. So "almost always" isn't good enough. "Always" has to be hardwired.

The government requires every hospital that receives government payment (Medicare or Medicaid) to administer and report these survey results. Beginning in 2013, hospital reimbursement will be based on value-based perfor-mance as HCAHPS moves from pay-for-reporting to pay-for-performance. As noted earlier, the new Patient Protection and Affordable Care Act signed into law in March 2010 also directs hospitals to collaborate with physicians in accountable care organizations for shared responsibility in meeting quality and cost savings.

But wait...there's even more good news. CG-CAHPS (Clinician and Group Consumer Assessment of Healthcare Providers Survey) is already be-ing reported by some practices on a voluntary basis. It is almost a certainty that this data will be ultimately available on an individual physician basis for all physicians. Your patients will be able to look at your practice and see how you perform in a variety of clinical scenarios.

It is my belief that in the early years of this project, there will be some dis-tinguishing characteristics between institutions, but I predict that eventually the spread will decrease as all institutions revert to the mean. In the interven-ing years, I know that my hospital and yours will focus a tremendous amount of effort on ensuring that we do not fall short in these measures.

With that in mind, it behooves you to understand what data is currently being reported about you and your organization, to ensure that you are not on the short end of the perceived quality stick. I do believe that once this all shakes out, quality will again be essentially equivalent across the board (though perhaps at an even higher standard) and have limited utility as a marketing tool.

Service, on the other hand, will always differentiate one practitioner from another. This, I believe, is where you can truly make a difference both in your own practice and in your patients' lives. My role as a surgeon is not merely to perform the highest quality operation and offer quality hospital care, but to provide care and comfort to patients and their families. This is where I believe I make a difference in people's lives, and my patients feel it, too.

Measuring Service

One way of measuring service is through patient satisfaction surveys. These are critical and useful tools, both as an internal measurement tool to create your superior service line and maintain it and also as an advertising tool to demonstrate your superiority in this arena to others. In the vocabulary of our Five Ps, patient satisfaction surveys can help you improve your positioning in the minds of your patients, and can also be used as a promotional tool.

Again, whether you know this or not, your hospital is measuring patient satisfaction on a large scale through a vendor that regularly surveys your patients. The HCAHPS questions are included on this survey and are publicly reported. Savvy hospitals are drilling down on these results to look at the performance of individual physicians. So, for example, if a hospital's scores are low on the "communication with doctors," questions, its leadership can find out which doctors are scoring poorly and suggest training to improve those doctors' results.

It is not the intent of this book to teach you how to manage your survey results. Just know that they are out there. To ensure your service scores are impeccable, I recommend you review some of the tools and techniques in *The HCAHPS Handbook*, written by a group of experts from outcomes firm Studer Group', and in Dr. Stephen Beeson's excellent book *Practicing Excellence*. Quint Studer's seminal books *Hardwiring Excellence* and *Straight A Lead-*

ership will also provide you and your organization with specific, time-tested methods for exceeding patient expectations.

Returning to general principles of marketing, creating a point of differentiation will serve you well as a strategy to grow and maintain your practice. Service is but one way to do this. You may have a certain niche that is otherwise unavailable in your area that makes you different from your competitors.

You may have a group of physicians with unique characteristics that allow you to position yourself in the marketplace. For example, a large group of female physicians have the potential to utilize that differentiator to their advantage. They can market themselves as a "Women's Health Center," if they wish to target that demographic. The same goes for ethnic groups, languages spoken, and many other individual features that may be a worthwhile selling point to your targeted audience.

Who Is Your Customer?

As we have been discussing your target market, we have clearly been referring to patients. However, depending on the nature of your practice, you may find that your business comes from sources other than patients themselves. For example, many specialists get most of their new patients from referring physicians. While most people don't know what a pediatric endocrinologist does, I know that a good pediatric endocrinologist is productive and busy all the time. That's in large part due to the referrals that doctor receives.

Where do her patients come from? I would venture to guess that they come mostly from pediatricians. So, if her target market is pediatricians, she needs to convince them that she is the pediatric endocrinologist of choice in her community. For others, large corporations—or insurance companies or hospital administrators—may provide their patient base. In any event, it is important to understand your practice's referral patterns and from whom your patients get your name, so you can nurture those relationships.

Advertising

Once you understand what your point of differentiation is and who your target markets are, then you can work on positioning. Here is where advertising comes in. In order to advertise, you first have to create a compelling message. Any advertising that you do should have the threefold goal of helping your "customer" (e.g., the patient, the referring doctor) to identify, understand, and remember the uniqueness you are trying to communicate. The message is most effective if it is simple. It would be great if it were enough to say "quality." But again, for the reasons stated above, that's just not going to work for any of us.

Think for a moment: What do you think of when you hear the word "Volvo"?

How many of you answered "style"? Just kidding. None of you did. I would bet that 99 percent of you reading the above question answered: "safety." That's no accident (pardon the pun). Volvo has spent decades honing their message of safety to the point where you, the target audience, think of nothing else when you think of Volvo. The simplicity and the power of that message are staggering. You would do well to find a message that so resonates with your patient base, referring physicians, or other target market.

Once you have created this message, you can then consider advertising. Remember the subway hemorrhoid guy? Well, times have changed quite a bit since then. While it is still not quite de rigueur for physicians to advertise their services, it has become much more commonplace and much less vulgar in appearance. Institutions and large clinical practices do it all the time. Individual physicians and small groups in certain areas are also becoming more aggressive in their advertising efforts.

Remember, there are a number of different ways in which to advertise. Typical forms of advertising include: direct mail, telephone listings (such as ads in the Yellow Pages), newspaper ads, magazine ads, radio and TV commercials, and signs. We will consider other forms of communicating your message in the following chapter, "How to Build a Practice."

One of the problems with advertising in traditional media is that it is just so expensive. And, as we learned in the previous section, you really need to be able to quantify the returns on investment in order to determine whether or not this is an effective use of your money. This can prove to be extremely difficult in the realm of advertising. How you track the results of any given ad or ad campaign is a matter of great debate and great uncertainty. Whatever you do, make sure that tracking—or at least a legitimate attempt at tracking—outcomes is a significant part of your advertising campaign. This will help you answer the all-important question: Is it worth it?

More Advanced Marketing and Strategic Planning

SWOT Analysis

Many mature businesses employ SWOT analysis to determine and articulate the internal and external factors and forces that contribute to or detract from their success. SWOT is an acronym for strengths, weaknesses, opportunities, and threats. The analysis is simple to perform and can be quite useful for an individual or a large multi-specialty practice. The analysis consists merely of a grid (see Figure 5.1) into which you list the various aspects in their appropriate quadrant. Strengths and weaknesses refer to internal factors, and opportunities and threats refer to external factors in the marketplace.

Figure 5.1: SWOT

Strengths	Weaknesses
Threats	Opportunities

In performing such an analysis, it pays to be brutally honest about your own strengths and weaknesses and to keep the grid as simple as possible. The point of this exercise is not necessarily to be able to create a detailed, strategic plan; however, the act of performing the exercise itself is often very revealing and can help to focus your efforts and your understanding of your place in the world.

An example of an ophthalmology practice's SWOT analysis appears in Figure 5.2.

Figure 5.2: SWOT Example: Ophthalmology Practice

Strengths	Weaknesses
• Most Subspecialties Covered • Updated Equipment • All Trained at Top Programs	• No Oculoplastics Practice • Out-of-the-Way Office • Dingy Space
Threats	**Opportunities**
• 3 Large Groups Within 5-Mile Radius • Commoditization of Laser Surgery • Declining Government Reimbursements	• Graduating Oculoplastics Fellow • New Office Space Available • Potential Insurance Contract with Large Employer

In this example, a large ophthalmology practice recognizes that although they have modern equipment and cover most specialties (their strengths), they are missing a segment of business in not having an oculoplastics practice. Additionally, they view their dingy office space as a point of weakness. As an opportunity, they list the possibility of rectifying one of these weaknesses by hiring a potentially available ocular plastics fellow. Additionally, there is new office space coming on the market that may be worth looking into.

External threats include three large groups that are within a five-mile radius, which compete for their business. The commoditization of laser surgery and surgeons makes it difficult to maintain a differential advantage in this setting. And, of course, declining reimbursement continues to be an external threat to this (and every) medical enterprise.

A great strategy employed by many businesses is to use their weaknesses and turn them into strengths. An example in consumer products is that of the Smucker's brand of jams and jellies. A SWOT analysis of the J.M. Smucker Company included its name as a weakness, and yet, I'm sure you are already reciting the tagline in your head: "With a name like Smucker's, it has to be good!"

For our ophthalmology group in the above example, certainly new office space and a better location might be a desirable solution. If that proves not to be feasible, then their positioning strategy may include a nod to this, something along the lines of, "Worth the search. Good doctors are hard to find."

This type of advertising was used quite effectively by the Mount Sinai Hospital in New York in the years following the September 11 attack. One of the large target markets for Mount Sinai has been patients who live in the suburbs of Manhattan in Long Island, Westchester, and New Jersey. For a while following September 11, 2001, patients were understandably reluctant to travel to New York City for medical care, as well as for the other activities that they had previously enjoyed in Manhattan.

But eventually people started coming back to New York, and Mount Sinai effectively advertised on the back cover of *Playbill Magazine*, which is given out to each audience member at on- and off-Broadway shows, and on the back cover of the game-day magazines given out at professional sporting events such as baseball games, hockey games, and basketball games. The tagline read, "If you can go into the city to see a show [game], you can go into the city to save your life."

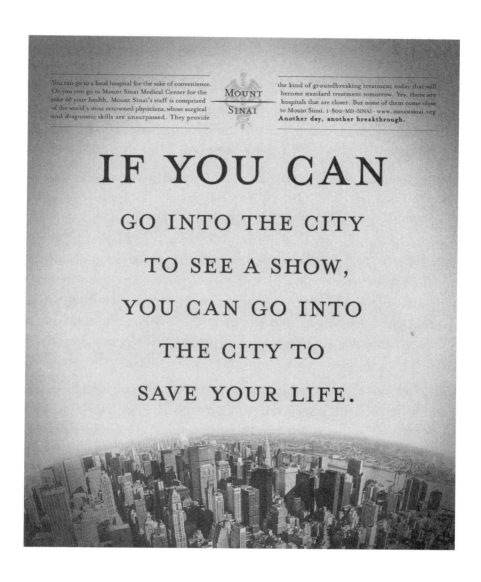

Once you have created a SWOT analysis, it is worth discussing with your management team or colleagues ways in which you might maximize strengths and opportunities and minimize weaknesses and threats. This is an exercise that is worth revisiting from time to time, as both internal and external market forces change.

Relationship Marketing

Relationship marketing is probably what most good doctors do best. Despite this, it also offers the most opportunity to improve and grow your practice. You are already practicing relationship marketing, I know, but it may be instructive to articulate what it is that you are doing.

In traditional marketing, the seller has a product or service that he is prepared to offer, he determines how best to position that product or service in order to reach the most potential customers, and he prices it in order to maximize his revenue and grow that business. Relationship marketing turns this paradigm on its head. In its purest sense, this market-based approach is best performed by first determining what it is that the customer wants (or more precisely, what the needs of the customer base are), then planning and developing the service (or product) that will meet those needs, and then determining the best way to provide that service or product. The best way to do this is to include the customer in one's decision making.

Again, I maintain that if you are reading this book, you already do this all the time. Each time you phone a referring physician's office, each time you give your business card to the registrar in the emergency room, each time you look at the calendar with a patient and her family to determine the best date for her surgery, you are, in a sense, using the tools of relationship marketing.

Let's go back to my radiology friend, to whom I briefly introduced you in the introduction for this section. You may remember that he had contacted me to discuss ways we might improve my patients' access to his services. This strategy had within it some real genius and had the potential to dramatically improve his business.

When I spoke with him, I asked him why he had contacted me rather than one of the other doctors. He told me two things: First, he said he was reviewing the volumes of his radiology practice and its referring physicians, and noticed that I sent almost no radiology business his way. Next, he said that as friends, he finds me very approachable, which was important since this can sometimes be an uncomfortable kind of phone call. This call to me was the first of what was to be many of his efforts to reach out to his referral base.

Here's the genius in this. First, he recognized that our friendship made me inclined to want to speak with him and certainly made it easier for him to practice his pitch.

Second, and more importantly, embedded in the offer was his distinct willingness to change the way he does business in order to accommodate me and my patients. This was huge.

He was trying to engage me in a process redesign of his business that would service my needs and therefore increase his volume.

The truly brilliant nature of this kind of strategy is in what happens down the line when it is employed. Once we have together created a strategy to streamline patient flow from my office to his, then the path of least resistance for me will be to send him all of my patients with radiology needs.

Let's look at his radiology practice for a second, as if it were a castle. His goal is to get as many people into his castle as possible—doctors or patients, really, whoever his target market is—by essentially lowering the drawbridge for easier entry. But in order to enter, a patient will need to exit across the drawbridge of another castle (e.g., a competitor's radiology practice).

In our metaphor here, my friend's drawbridge is essentially, in marketing terms, a "barrier to entry." By reaching out to me, and trying to make it easy for me to bring patients his way, he is lowering the barrier of entry for my referrals. A prime example of that in medicine is the practice of sending transportation to patients' homes, or to referring doctors' offices, in order to deliver patients to your practice or hospital.

On the other side of this, as well, my radiology buddy is simultaneously raising his "barrier to exit." By having me design a process that is, by default, easier than sending patients to any other radiology practice, he has created a more difficult task for me to go back to his competitors. This is, all in all, a brilliant strategy—one that you should think about very seriously. Think about your barriers to entry and your barriers to exit and how you can lower the former and raise the latter. We will talk more about this in the chapter on loyalty.

Unfortunately, this particular phone call was not at all fruitful for my colleague. He is not likely to see a single additional patient by reaching out to me. And why is that? Remember, I sent virtually no patients to his practice. That can mean one of two things: Either I already have a strong relationship with one or more other radiology practices, or I don't use radiology services at all. Either way, I am not likely to be the best use of his resources in trying to grow his business. Either I'm just a bad prospect, or the barrier to exit from my current radiologist is too high.

So I suggested an alternative strategy in selecting his next set of phone calls. I told him to look at his referral numbers and break them down into three groups. Group 1, which includes me, are those physicians with extremely low utilization of his services. Group 2 are those physicians who use him some of the time, but who clearly, based on the types of practices that they have, are using other radiologists as well. And Group 3 are those very high-volume referrers who seem to be using his group as their primary, if not exclusive, radiology practice. I recommended he use a different marketing strategy for each of these groups.

Group 1—the low utilization group—should be ignored. There is little value in attempting to change someone's mind completely when he is so entrenched somewhere else. You can try, and you might even be successful, but it would likely require an overwhelming campaign and excessive utilization of resources that would not be warranted by the yield that you could expect. It would be akin to the Pepsi people trying to get me to stop drinking Diet Coke (not ever going to happen).

Group 3—the high volume referrers—is easier. He already has them, and his job is to keep them. I suggested that he reach out to them in a manner that reflects his humility and gratefulness that these practices are sending all of their radiology work to him and his group. I suggested that he ask them if everything is okay and if there would be anything that he could do to make their lives a little easier—in other words, to raise the barrier to exit.

It is this middle group, Group 2 (the part-time users), where my friend's efforts can have the most impact. Clearly, in this group are physicians who don't seem to have a particular preference as to where their patients go, perhaps because they find all groups to be essentially equal in their minds. To this group, radiologists are a commodity. It is for this group that this type of call can have the most impact by differentiating his service. He can reduce the barrier to entry for patients from these practices and increase his own barriers to exit at the same time. He can do this by asking the physicians and/or the staff members in the physicians' offices to help him redesign his patient flow process to make it easier and better for them. He can create for them the "wow experience" that engenders increased customer satisfaction and, as a result, loyalty and greater market share.

Although I personally was not going to be a source of significant new business to my friend, I am certain that our discussion will have a huge impact on his strategic planning efforts.

Key Learning Points: Marketing Is Not Advertising

1. Marketing includes differentiating yourself from your competition and understanding your position in the minds of your target market. Understand the "Five Ps" of marketing: product, price, place, promotion, and positioning.

2. Quality is the price of entry in healthcare today, and, therefore, not likely to be particularly useful (for long) as a marketing tool. Visit the CMS website, hospitalcompare.hhs.gov, today to see how your hospital stacks up.

3. Service is, and will always be, a strong differentiator among physician practices. Ensure that patient perception of your care is excellent.

4. Know your customer. In addition to your patients, pay particular attention to referral patterns from specialists and other physicians. Nurture key relationships.

5. Advanced marketing tactics include: (a) using SWOT analysis and (b) harnessing the power of relationship marketing.

CHAPTER 6
HOW TO BUILD A PRACTICE
· · · · · · · · · · ·

If you are going to read only one chapter of this book, this is the chapter to read.

In this chapter we will discuss the specific ways in which you can use the tools of marketing and strategic planning that we discussed in Chapter 5—in particular, positioning and relationship marketing—to build and grow your practice and reputation.

We will look at techniques and specific strategies to use for your referrers, patients, employees, and staff; we will explore ways to enhance your position and reputation; and we will conclude by looking at a special situation, which is that of how to incorporate a junior partner into your practice, including insurance strategies around practice expansion. I believe that all of these subjects are equally relevant whether you are just starting out in practice or if you have been successful in your practice for the past 30 years.

Referring Physicians: A Key Relationship

Depending on your situation, the term "referring physician" may be too narrow or flat out misleading. I am using this term here to specify whoever it is who first tells the patients about who you are and why they should see you.

In many, if not most, doctors' practices, this group mainly consists of referring physicians. However, in other cases, this term can refer to large employers, union health plans, or HMOs.

This group, in my opinion, is the highest value target for strategically building your practice. Referring physicians (and their equivalents) hold the key to your potential for explosive growth or, as we shall see in the next chapter, the death of your medical or surgical practice. This is the group that requires the greatest attention for most specialists, in terms of strategic planning and marketing efforts. There are some exceptions, of course, in which self-referral is a larger source of business, but I would venture to bet that for most of you, the real heart of your practice lies here.

Because my staff knows this, they use particular rules for managing calls from referring physicians. Calls are broken down into four categories. In ascending order of urgency, they are: (1) a high-volume referrer calling about an established patient; (2) a new physician calling about an established patient; (3) a high-volume referrer calling about a new patient; and (4) the highest priority, which is a new referrer calling about a new patient. My staff knows that for such a call, they are to track me down, wherever I am, confirm with me that they have reached me, and make sure that I return that phone call immediately.

Of course, this is not to say that I ignore any of my phone calls. Quite the opposite. My referring physicians know that as soon as it is reasonably possible (almost always within a couple of hours), I will return their calls, and that if there is an emergency, they can reach me immediately. But a new doctor calling about a new patient requires a different level of response.

Why is that? Let's go back to the concept of relationship marketing that we just discussed. Clearly, this new referring physician would not be calling me if he were completely satisfied with the surgical care his patients have been receiving from other surgeons.

Somewhere there is a chink in the armor. The barrier to exiting the other practice he usually refers to is suddenly lower for some reason. My job is to lower my barrier to entry to such a degree as to capture this and potential future business from this referring physician. An immediate response, which harkens back to our three A's (Affable, Able, and Available), begins that process.

What Do Referring Physicians Want?

The more accurately and completely that you can answer this question, the more successful you will be at meeting their needs. This is relationship marketing at its finest. In my experience, there are several universal themes to the wants and needs of physicians referring their patients to other specialists.

First, they want great clinical outcomes for their patients. Of course, as I showed you in Chapter 5, this is a given, and your ability to use this as a point of differentiation is essentially zero. However, you must provide consistently great outcomes as a baseline. Otherwise, you need to look for another line of work.

Second, like their patients, these physicians want you to relieve their anxiety. In many cases, there is some uncertainty about the aforementioned outcome at the time in which the physician is referring the patient to you. Both the patient and the referring physician feel that anxiety. It is your job to relieve it.

Third, the referring doctor wants her patient's experience with you to reflect well on her. You can help her strengthen her relationship with the patient by "managing up" the referring physician when you see the patient. "You are so fortunate to have Dr. Davis as your primary care physician," you might say. "We have worked together for a number of years now and I find her to be an outstanding physician." Never make it up—share something you find to be true about the physician.

I find that when physicians manage each other up, everybody wins. The patient is grateful to the referring physician for directing him to you; the referring physician appreciates your positive words; and perhaps most importantly, this reinforces the seamless continuity of care that patients truly appreciate.

On one occasion, I was on speakerphone with one of my most precious referral sources, who had also become a close friend. He was in the car with his precocious five-year-old son, who asked who was on the phone. I said, "Hi, it's Mickey Harris." He said, "Oh, I know you. You're daddy's surgical instrument."

We were hysterically laughing, and now, years later, continue to laugh about that incident. But it was perfect. Every patient that he refers to me goes back to this gastroenterologist and commends him on his use of me as his surgical instrument. I have done a great job in managing a source of enormous future business. I want him to look brilliant every time he uses my name.

Next, the referring doctors want you to make their lives easier. Again, the advice I was given when I first joined the practice—to act like an owner, not a renter—has been particularly useful. (When you own your home, you mow the lawn and make needed repairs to protect your investment. When you rent a home, you wait for someone else to fix it.) The more that I can do to relieve the burden and responsibility for any particular issue from the mind of the referring physician, the better I have served him.

During my residency, one of my senior residents, a guy whom I respected tremendously, gave me a couple of words of advice. He said, "There are only three words that are acceptable for you to say when being given an instruction by somebody senior to you. Those words are, 'Done. What else?'"

I highly recommend that phrase as a starting point in practice building. You should allow your referring physician to feel that he can wash his hands of any issues that might arise during your tenure as a specialist in the care of a particular patient, even if your specialty is primary care.

As we discussed earlier, you are a specialist, too. But whether your referral base is a group of physicians, an insurance company, an employer, or a community, the referrer wants to know that patients are safe in your hands and that you will take ownership for ensuring all goes well.

Another thing that referring doctors want is to have their patients return to them after your treatment episode has concluded. An example: Nothing is more infuriating to a gastroenterologist than to send a patient to a surgeon, only to have that surgeon refer the patient to another gastroenterologist for follow-up. It shows a lack of gratitude for the referral and a profound lack of respect for the referring physician. Keep this in mind as you navigate the waters of a patient's experience.

The referral chain is not always straightforward. The GYN oncologist who referred the patient to your radiation oncology practice probably was initially referred by an OB/GYN or primary care physician. Before you call the dermatologist to help manage the skin irritation that is a side effect of your therapy, pause for a moment.

Is this the physician that the patient's own doctor would call upon? There is power and money in referrals, so demonstrate respect and courtesy for your referring physician by checking about her dermatologist preference before you make a referral. Even better, ask your referring doctor if she would prefer to make that call. And make sure that the patient returns to that original physician who referred her patient to you.

Tools to Use in Serving Referring Physicians

Here are some of the tools that you can use to serve your referring physicians. You will note that virtually all of these fall under the realm of communication.

USE THE TELEPHONE!

While in our digital age, email and text messaging are often excellent means of communicating with referring physicians, nothing beats an actual conversation. Of course, a face-to-face conversation trumps all. Do not assume that the referring doctor either knows what is going on at any given time, or does not care to know what is going on.

COMMUNICATE FREQUENTLY.

In my practice, there are a number of events—or "touch points" in relationship marketing—that automatically trigger phone calls to referring doctors. First, as I review my schedule for upcoming office hours (which I do religiously at least 48 hours in advance), I will call the referring physician for any new patient I see on my schedule.

This has a variety of beneficial effects. First, when you do this, you assure the referring doctor that the patient has, in fact, followed up on her recommendations and made an appointment to see you. Second, it alleviates some of her anxiety in making that referral in the first place. She knows that you are paying attention and are serious about her patient—so much so that you have taken the time to learn as much as you can in advance of the patient's visit.

Third, it allows you to say to the patient, when you greet him, that you have spoken to his referring physician and that the two of you have spent some time thinking about ways to optimize the value of this visit and best coordinate his care. This alleviates the patient's anxiety and elevates both you and the referring physician in the patient's estimation. It also prevents errors. It allows you to ensure that you do, in fact, have the appropriate information prior to the patient's visit.

FOLLOW UP AFTER THE INITIAL VISIT.

Make a second phone call to the referring physician after the initial visit to again thank the referrer for her confidence in you. Recap the results of your consultation. Because it is not always completely clear what the next steps should be in a patient's care, this gives you an opportunity to get feedback from the referring doctor before going forward. In addition, it further alleviates the referring physician's anxiety and uncertainty, and allows her to continue to participate in the plan. She also is subtly reassured that the patient is still hers.

HARDWIRE OFFICE-TO-OFFICE COMMUNICATION.

The next call is from my office to her office. Once a plan is established (especially if it includes the patient's being admitted and/or undergoing surgery), my office will inform the referring physician's office about the specific date and time of any upcoming intervention. This allows for the referring physician's staff to put this on her calendar. Additionally, it creates an office-to-office communication that can be extremely useful in patient care. Typically, this is the second interaction between my office and hers. The first will have been when the patient initially makes an appointment and my office contacts them for medical records and/or other information.

CALL POST-OP.

The next physician-to-physician call occurs when the patient is operated upon (or any other intervention is performed). And I mean right after the operation. The last thing you would want is for the patient's family member to catch the referring physician unaware of what occurred in the OR. This also gives me an opportunity to speak with the physician's office staff, who are often as anxious about the outcome of the surgery as is the referring doctor.

CALL ABOUT COMPLICATIONS.

In my practice, many referring physicians are daily visitors to our post-operative patients because they work in the same hospital. Others, however, are not doctors at my hospital, and require a higher frequency of telephone conversation. In any event, any complication should automatically trigger a call. Again, there is nothing more embarrassing to a doctor than to hear from a family member what she should already know about a patient's condition.

I cannot stress this enough. How you manage complications, both in terms of your communication with the patient and his family, as well as communication with referring physicians, says more about you as a physician and an individual than almost any other interpersonal interaction.

Part of your "positioning" should be that you are a stand-up individual. Where I come from, it's called being a mensch, which the dictionary defines as "a decent, responsible person with admirable characteristics."

CALL UPON DISCHARGING THE PATIENT.

The next call to the referring physician is on discharge. Again, this reinforces the notion that you are returning the patient to the care of his physician. Additionally, it lets her know what has transpired during the hospital stay.

SEND A LETTER.

Another enormously important communication tool is a letter. The younger of you may not recognize this term. It is kind of like an email, only using actual paper and ink and sent through the U.S. mail. Do not underestimate its value. First, letters are an excellent documentation tool. Particularly in the day of the electronic medical record, where data are stored in ways that tend to be more and more templated, a good old-fashioned letter can sometimes tell the story best. Additionally, there is still something elegant and charming about a well-worded communication on fine stationery. To me, this is an expense that is well-justified. Thirdly, there is the very real potential to get more business from a fortuitously timed referral or follow-up letter.

Imagine a cardiologist in his office hours. He is seeing an inordinate number of patients in the hopes of fighting his diminishing income from declining reimbursements. His day is somewhat frenzied, as you can imagine. In between his 10- or 15-minute patient slots, he is trying to eat his lunch, manage his practice, review patient results, and make phone calls. He just got a follow-up letter from you stating that Mrs. Jones's hemoglobin A1c is now under excellent control. It's still sitting on his desk. Lo and behold, Mr. Thomas comes in, who requires help managing his diabetes. Whom do you think the cardiologist is going to call? Don't laugh. I promise you I have received many referrals as a direct result of this happy accident.

At the end of the day, the key to managing your referring physicians is to think like them, to try to discern what it is that they want and need, and to provide it for them. In addition to that, if you can subtly make sure they know that this is what you are doing, you have done your job well.

Exceed Your Patients' Expectations

The above principles are essentially unchanged when applied to patients as well. Patients thrive on communication. When we apply our concept of relationship marketing to patients, and attempt to define what they want and need, virtually all of their needs and desires are met by the doctor who excels in his communication skills. Studies qualitatively and quantitatively define what patients are looking for in a physician. You might be surprised to learn that patients' ratings of their doctors are almost never associated with the technical quality of their care. Rather, they are always associated with the level of communication.[5]

Of course, patients want their doctors to be competent, but they assume that to be the case. What they are looking for is to be cared for by someone who respects their concerns and alleviates their fear and anxiety. It has also been well-documented that communication leads to better patient compliance and improved outcomes. Many excellent books have been written on this subject. (I again refer you to Studer Group's books in the Fire Starter Publishing family. You can browse them at FireStarterPublishing.com.)

Use AIDET

If you are not familiar with the concept of AIDET^SM, you should be. At first blush, to the doctor with an edge, the concept may appear hokey, but when you break it down into its components, as we have in the figure below, you quickly realize that each piece of this is critical, and that the acronym can focus your conversation in order to create a desired connection with a patient and her family.

A	is for *acknowledge:* greeting patients and establishing a first impression
I	is for *introduce:* introducing physicians and others to patients, explaining their roles on the care team, and outlining the experience and expertise they bring to the case
D	is for *duration:* keeping patients informed on wait times, admission length, test turnaround times, therapeutic effect, or symptom resolution
E	is for *explanation:* providing patients with information on treatment, medications, diagnosis, and therapy options
T	is for *thank you:* thanking patients for trusting physicians with their care as well as closing the clinical encounter

Adapted from materials prepared by Studer Group.®
Copyright 2010, Studer Group, All Rights Reserved, Used with Permission.

There is no question that most of us cover most of the components of AIDET in most of our conversations, but that is just not good enough. Remember HCAHPS, which we discussed back in Chapter 5? Our goal is to hardwire a culture of always. Every patient every time. The beauty of AIDET is that it ensures you are extremely consistent. Do not worry about sounding scripted. You will find very quickly that you have created your own language and tone around each of the five areas, and soon it will become a natural part of your conversation. (To learn more about AIDET, visit StuderGroup.com.)

An example might sound like this:

"Hi, my name is Mickey Harris. I've been a surgeon at Mount Sinai for 22 years and specialize in caring for people with Crohn's disease. I work with Dr. George all the time, and we have already spoken about you—he has been taking great care of you. I'd like to spend the next 10 to 15 minutes talking about what's been happening with you, and then we'll go into the other room, where I'll take a quick look at your belly. That should take only a few minutes. Then we'll come back here, and I'll review all of your options and help you decide which is the best one for you. I'll answer all of your questions and make sure that you understand everything before you leave. The whole visit should take about an hour."

At the end of the visit: "It was a pleasure meeting you. Thank you for coming in to see me."

(This took me 22 seconds to say. And that was speaking really slowly.)

I find that the more complete and detailed the initial conversation is with the patient and his family, the less time is spent, in the long run, re-explaining and rehashing issues.

In my own practice, it is the pre-operative discussion that holds the key. I am sure there is a similar moment in your relationship with your patients where this applies. I spend an inordinate amount of time with patients discussing what their expectations should be, both in the short- and the long-term. Actually, I focus on the long-term outcomes first. I always make sure that I cover the "D" and the "E" of AIDET.

I tend to use drawings, which I create anew, in each discussion. Sure, I could use either prefabricated drawings or illustrations, or I could even use one that I had used before so many, many times. But I find that it is helpful to create a drawing for a patient, and the patients love it. They feel that the act of drawing their anatomy and their issues focuses me and ensures that I am speaking only of them and not speaking in abstract terms about generic patients.

Recently, a new patient, who is an educator at a large university, commended me on my teaching skills. I found that to be very flattering and thought it an apt way to describe the conversations that I have with my patients. There is clearly an aspect of teaching involved in helping to bring the patient and his family to your level of understanding of his condition and your expectations going forward.

To create a genuine and personal relationship with a patient who will remain loyal to you, never be condescending or use medical jargon without explaining what you mean. Patients can sniff out arrogance and condescension quicker than you can imagine, and this will send them to your competitors. I can tell you it is quite rare for a patient to see me in consultation and then be operated on by someone else. Try drawing pictures. There is a quaintness about it and also a bit of self-deprecation involved, particularly if you are (as I am) a horrendous artist.

Embrace Technology That Brings You Closer to Patients

If you really want to take it to a higher level, there is a new technology that I recently discovered that you may want to review. Check out Livescribe.com. This company has created a pen and special paper that records both voice and pen strokes concomitantly and provides the ability to play back both the conversation and the movement of the pen on a computer screen. Additionally, it allows the user to point the pen on the paper or the cursor on the screen to a certain part of the page, at which time the conversation recorded, at that moment, will be replayed.

The husband of a patient shared this with me as I was discussing the results of his wife's surgery with him. He sent me an email of the conversation, which was truly amazing. I have not yet come to use this for all of my pre-operative discussions, but it's certainly something to think about. (See an example at FireStarterPublishing.com/ExcellenceWithAnEdge.)

Some of you might also like to use handouts, brochures, or other printed materials in lieu of or in addition to drawings in your pre-operative discussion or its equivalent. I think in many cases this is an excellent idea.

For example, I recently coached a neurosurgeon on improving his communication with patients and suggested just such a solution. His patients reported difficulty understanding his language (he has a heavy foreign accent) and were frustrated with his inability to spend enough time with them. For someone like this, pre-printed explanations and drawings of the procedures he commonly performs may enhance communication and reduce anxiety on both sides. Since he has made this change, his patient satisfaction has improved dramatically.

Some Other Thoughts on Communicating with Patients

In general, remember that the major initial discussion is a conversation between people. Do not underestimate your patients' intelligence. Do not underestimate their ability to understand complex issues. Do not talk down to them. Educate them, yes, but demonstrate your respect for them and for their ability to comprehend what you are explaining. And then stop and make sure that they, in fact, did understand, by asking leading questions to confirm that this is the case.

Follow-up phone calls are critical, particularly in complex or high-anxiety situations. In addition to reducing patient anxiety, these calls reduce complaints and malpractice claims, reinforce the patient's perception that excellent care has been provided, and offer an opportunity for quick service recovery.

Research shows that there is a direct correlation between the quality of discharge planning and readmission to the hospital. In addition, follow-up phone calls improve patient satisfaction and reduce medication-related problems.[6] In one survey[7] of 400 patients, 19 percent had suffered an adverse event after discharge—nearly one in five patients! Some other food for thought: 48 percent of these were preventable. And the vast majority were adverse drug events.

It does not take a great deal of effort to call a patient a day or two after you have seen her to say, "I'm just calling to follow up and make sure that you fully understood everything we spoke about. I also wanted to see if any additional questions came up." Ask if she has filled her prescription or has any problems with her medication that would keep her from complying with your instructions.

Three things will happen when you make such a call. First, the patient will be amazed and truly grateful that you made the call. It will confirm to her that you are indeed the mensch that she thought you were. Next, it will allow her to clarify something that has been nagging at her for the couple of days since you saw her.

In my experience, this call never generates more than one or two questions. You do not need to fear that the entire office conversation will need to be repeated. You also do not need to worry that your effort to reach out will be misinterpreted by patients as an open invitation to contact you frequently with inconsequential questions and concerns. While there may be an occasional unreasonable patient who does engage in such behavior—and you should gently re-set his expectations in such a case—I find that the majority of patients do not abuse such access.

Third, and equally important, you will have, for lack of a more graceful term, "completed the sale." Particularly in the type of environment in which we practice, where patients will frequently seek multiple opinions, you will differentiate yourself from your peers by following up in this way. Quite frankly, post-visit phone calls also reduce late-night phone calls into the practice.

A word of caution here, though. Make sure that the call is, in fact, in the spirit of continuing to comfort and care for the patient. A colleague of mine is known for making similar post-visit phone calls to patients considering surgery. However, I have been told many times by patients on whom I have subsequently consulted that this physician's calls were transparent attempts to get the patient to lock in a date for surgery that he was not quite sure he was ready to undergo.

Making after-care phone calls is the right thing to do. Intuitively I know this as I have called every single patient on whom I have operated in the last 17 years within 48 hours of his or her discharge from the hospital. And again, the response from the patients is overwhelmingly positive when I tell them that I'm just calling to check up on them to make sure that they're okay at home, and to see if they have any questions or concerns.

My last bit of advice about phone calls is a simple but inviolate rule: Always return every phone call, no matter what, on the same day. It is never too late. The response you will hear, which never ceases to amaze me, is, "Thank you so much for calling me back." I'm not sure that I really understand that. Clearly there must be many, many physicians out there who don't answer their phone calls or don't call patients back on the same day. Besides being the wrong thing to do, it is also bad for business.

What About Email?

Many physicians understandably choose to communicate with their patients via email. This may provide a level of access and service that is desirable for their practice and their target markets of referring physicians and patients. I, however, prefer the telephone or, as I said before, face-to-face conversation.

I find it is often difficult to convey the proper emotion or tone in an email. (I believe you would find me more charming in person than the snarky tone in this book might suggest! If you could hear my voice, you would be smiling rather than shaking your head.) Something else to consider: Privacy and other potential legal implications are currently being debated with regard to the use of email in clinical settings.

Include Patient Families in Your Communications

Part of communication with patients is communicating with their loved ones as well. Most patients in typical situations, whether complex or anxiety-provoking, will bring a parent or spouse or friend to participate in the conversation. I welcome this, and you should, too.

In fact, studies have shown that engaging each and every member of a patient's entourage individually and personally will tremendously impact the patient's perception of his care. And in highly complex situations, particularly where there is the chance for major complications, having established a relationship with the patient's family or significant others sets the stage for your ability to work with them should the patient become temporarily or permanently incapacitated.

Communicate Proactively about Complications

This brings me to another important piece of relationship management advice. Be honest and completely forthright when dealing with untoward events. Bad things unfortunately happen, even when everything is done correctly. Hopefully, some of the shock of a complication will have been mitigated by the completeness of the pre-op discussion that you had at the first meeting.

In fact, all of your interactions with the patient and his family will have set the stage for your ability to communicate with him or his family when something has gone awry. Be straight, be honest, be complete, and be sorry, even if being sorry is not an admission of wrongdoing. If you have children, you will understand this last point.

Tell me if this interaction is familiar to you. Your six-year-old daughter is running outside and trips and falls down and bangs her knee. She's sitting on the ground crying, and you say to her, "What happened?" And she says, "I hurt my knee." And your response is, of course, "Oh, I'm sorry, honey." To which she will respond, almost invariably, "It's not your fault." But she still appreciates that you're sorry.

This is not too different from an interaction with a patient and his family when a complication has occurred. Sometimes physicians are concerned that if they say they are sorry, this will be construed as some type of admission of responsibility, thereby increasing the likelihood that they may be sued for malpractice. Studies show just the opposite. What patients most value in such situations is empathy and compassion from the physician. Malpractice is predicted by the degree to which communication has broken down.[8]

The other part of this conversation is an action plan. The patient and his family will lose confidence in you very quickly if you are able to point out a complication, but are unable to outline a plan of action. In this respect, it is not much different from the initial conversation, where the patient has a problem, not of your creation, and where you have the means, the ability, and the wherewithal to create a plan to help that patient. In the setting of a complication, there is merely a new starting point, and you should be able to articulate that plan, as well. A new set of drawings may, in fact, be helpful here.

And, as a reminder, be sure to communicate immediately with the referring physician as well. Be prepared to answer phone calls, spend additional time, express your empathy, and yet be focused on the plan of action. Untoward events are a time to engage more fully—not to become defensive, disengage, and disappear. That is where lawsuits are born, and reputations are ruined.

Building Your Reputation

It is worth reviewing here other methods of practice building besides your direct relationships with your referring physicians and patients and their families. There are a variety of opportunities in any practice setting to promote your services and to enhance your reputation and good name. One avenue, which is open to all physicians, is in the realm of science.

Regardless of your practice setting, your ability to perform even the simplest of clinical research is ever present. Even a "lowly" case report can give you an avenue to present a paper, give a talk, or meet new people in your field. In any environment, people are interested in what you do, particularly if you can make it interesting for them. Giving talks to a variety of different groups will enhance your reputation and get you business. There are numerous venues for this.

There are opportunities to give talks to nurses, students, hospital administrators, and members of other specialties, all within your own institution. Your community has local church or temple groups, community organizations, and charity groups that are potentially excellent outlets for giving talks. Additionally, the local chapters of your specialty societies are venues for involvement. These talks do not need to be terribly sophisticated in order to be effective. Sometimes simple is better.

For example, I recently gave a 30-minute breakfast talk to the nurses on the surgical floor on which many of my patients recuperate. We talked specifically about the anatomy of the operations that their patients have undergone, and about the reasons for and the management of tubes and drains that many of the patients have in the first several days after surgery. I cannot tell you how amazing the response was from this seemingly simple talk. The nurses stated that nobody ever took the time to explain any of this to them.

This was great all around. First, my patients are now being cared for by people who have a better understanding of what it is that they are doing. Second, this has resulted in an even better esprit de corps between the nurses and me. And third, these nurses have family members, friends, and others within their circle who are going to need surgery for inflammatory bowel disease. Whom do you think they are going to recommend?

Beyond talks and papers, we all have the opportunity to become involved in our specialty societies. Your involvement can be beneficial in a number of ways. First, it ensures that you keep abreast of new technology and advances in your particular field. Next, I have found that all of the specialty societies offer specialty-specific business education as part of their curricula, even if it is only in how to ensure proper billing and coding. And last, involvement in these societies can enhance your reputation within the field. By serving in a variety of volunteer positions, for example, you will make contacts and learn information that will offer you a distinct competitive advantage.

Granted, you are unlikely to get a significant amount of business from a group that mainly consists of your competitors; however, you should not underestimate the value of maintaining a good name within this group.

You will probably get the occasional patient referral from someone who practices in a different region from you. (I often see patients who got my name from a colleague of mine in Boston or L.A. or Chicago.)

Additionally, if you can rise through the ranks of leadership in your specialty society, you can establish a regional or national reputation that will enhance your status at home, in terms of your internal, institutional status and also in the potential for academic advancement in your medical school.

Get Involved in Your Own Organization

The real payoff, however, is getting involved in your own organization, whether it be your large multi-specialty medical group or the hospital at which you admit patients. Getting involved in the political and administrative structure of your institution affords a huge number of advantages to you in your practice.

My earliest exposure to politics came to me around the dinner table as a kid growing up in the late '60s and early '70s. My older sister frequently engaged with my parents in what I will gently describe as "heated political discourse." Of course, I was naïve—I was only ten—but even then, I believed that politics was something that I would be able to remain above. And even still later, at the end of my surgical training, I failed to see the hospital as a highly charged political environment.

But when I ultimately learned the reality of how a hospital actually functions as a community of many thousands, I embraced it, along with its inevitably political nature. I suggest you do the same.

First, in its purest sense, your involvement can have a real effect on your own environment and can afford you a great deal of control. This harkens back to my point in Chapter 1 where we discussed the "victim mentality" and the need to eliminate that from our mindset. Involvement in your organization's administrative and political structure allows you to exert control over your environment to make the greatest possible positive impact for you and your patients.

Along those lines, you will also find yourself in a position to avoid surprises that may affect your practice environment. You will hear things and note things before they happen and certainly before your competitors do. This will allow you to plan and act well in advance of your competition, creating a significant competitive advantage. Involvement in this arena can also be quite satisfying in and of itself. It is just one more way to feel a sense of purpose, worthwhile work, and making a difference in the lives of many.

As I noted earlier, I personally find that I truly enjoy (and seem to be fairly good at) this aspect of "medical practice." (My hospital's Executive Medical Board meeting is one of the highlights of my week.) While it is clearly not for everyone, I have found here a niche that has opened a number of doors for potential second career opportunities including, indirectly, my ability to write and publish this book.

Lastly, involvement in hospital politics is just good business. Once again, it opens you up to a market of potential patients and referrers that might otherwise be closed to you. In a large organization, such as the one where I practice, you can earn a reputation as a "reasonable man" among your colleagues that will serve you well in differentiating your practice from those of other physicians.

Additionally, my hospital involvement has exposed me to a variety of non-medical people who are involved at a philanthropic and/or Board of Trustees level with the institution. If you think about it from a marketing point of view, what better target market than the rich and powerful in the city in which you live and work?

I have cared for countless high-value, high-profile, and highly grateful patients who have contributed to the institution where I work by way of philanthropy. And it works in numerous directions. Do not underestimate the value of bringing philanthropic dollars to your hospital or medical school. Your patients benefit. Medical students benefit. Your reputation benefits.

Cultivate a Close Relationship with Your Staff

Your ability to enhance your reputation and that of your practice through relationship development is not limited to those outside of your own walls. Your employees and staff will also play an enormous role in both establishing and projecting your message of excellence to the outside world. We will discuss the issues of staff loyalty in Chapter 8, but for now, suffice it to say that how you treat the people with whom you work will be observed and noted not only by the staff members themselves, but also by your patients and your referring physicians.

It is well established that patient satisfaction is enhanced (or reduced) in great measure by the interaction between the physician and his staff. Additionally, employees' feelings of respect (or disdain) for you are clearly projected in their conversations with patients, other offices, and, of course, their own families and friends in their outside lives.

A happy employee can herself create a steady stream of new patients into your practice. In fact, you can probably use this as a litmus test for your own practice. Do your employees ask your opinion about medical matters? Do they periodically ask you to see friends or family members? If not, then you may want to examine your relationship with them and/or the nature of your practice.

Work Closely with Your Nurses and Residents

In the hospital setting, the same holds true of nurses, and in teaching hospitals, residents or house officers. The importance of these two groups of colleagues cannot be overstated. Not only do they, too, have friends and family who frequently request referrals for the best physicians for themselves, they often have the ability to direct patients within the system to one physician or another. Residents, in particular, can be a long-term source of referrals to you.

First, residents within your own specialty are bound to either move to other regions or to practice in a niche that might be slightly different from yours. The more freely you have given of your time and expertise, the greater your reputation with these physicians and the more likely they are to view you as a mentor to whom patients should be directed. It is also, of course, worthwhile to participate in the education of those specialists who are entering a field that is a natural referral base for you in your field.

Nurses, too, have a great ability to influence your practice in many ways. They, of course, are the ones who spend the most time with your hospitalized patients. While you may round on patients once or even twice a day, spending several minutes with them at each encounter, the nurses are there continuously. And while we teach all of our nurses to "manage up" the institution and the patient's physicians, those of you whom the nurses truly love and respect will clearly benefit from extra doses of managing up by the nursing staff.

As an aside, I encourage you to celebrate, on a regular basis, the value that your nurses bring to the care of your patients. Express appreciation often in person, to their supervisors, and in public forums. (Remember, behavior that is rewarded and recognized gets repeated!) Some of the best "doctors" I have ever met are nurses, and I am fortunate to work with them every day. Letting them know this not only enhances your reputation but also makes your life much easier.

I actually learned this last point on the first day of my internship in 1988. On July 1, I nervously exited the elevator on the unit to which I had been assigned. This was, of course, back in the "days of the giants," when there were two interns for about 40 patients and we took every other night call. My first encounter was with the charge nurse. I don't know what possessed me to say this, but it turned out to be one of the smartest things I ever did. I pulled her aside, and said:

"Hi. My name is Mickey, and I'm your new intern. As you must know, I have no idea what I am doing, but I know that you have been here a while and you, more than anybody, know what's going on, so just tell me what to do, and I'll do it. And hopefully I will learn something, and eventually I'll be useful in helping you take care of our patients."

I had two great months on that floor. I was actually able to get some sleep on the old, broken-down couch in the lounge. (I still have the scar in my right flank from where the spring was pressed into my skin.) Every morning at about five, one of the nurses would come in with the chart rack and a cup of coffee, gently wake me up, and say:

"Here's what's going on..." And she would proceed to go through the list of patients on the floor and pre-wire me for morning rounds.

It is amazing how helpful these professionals can be if you treat them with the respect and gratitude that they so clearly deserve.

Add a Junior Partner

So you're doing reasonably well, you're busy, and you're looking for ways to expand your practice. It's time to consider bringing on a junior partner. You've done the math, you've performed the blue sky analysis, and financially it appears to make sense. If done right, the addition of a junior partner can be an enormously successful strategy in building your medical practice—one that can yield expansion for years and decades to come. On the other hand, if not handled correctly, the addition of a junior partner can be a tremendous source of dissatisfaction and prove to be quite harmful to the reputation of a successful practice.

The first thing to do is to ensure you hire the right partner. Your goal is to select a physician whose conduct, behavior, and clinical performance are consistent with the standards and aspirations of your medical practice. Other than by selecting one of your own trainees, the best way to match physician candidates to your existing team is to develop a standardized process for physician interviews that will predict consistent success.

Behavior-based questions are particularly important because they can reveal an applicant's attitudes with respect to teamwork, leadership, caring and compassion, collaboration, communication, judgment, and problem solving. This approach also has the benefit of providing an effective apples-to-apples method of comparing the pool of applicants and reducing subjectivity in selection. (You can learn more at StuderGroup.com. Search on "Physician Selection Toolkit.")

Once he joins your practice, your interaction with your new partner will have a great effect on his reputation, as well as yours and that of your practice. Reputation, of course, translates into volume and revenues.

First, it is vital that you and your partner be seen together throughout the practice environment, whether it is in the office or the hospital or both. You want both patients and colleagues to envision the two (or more) of you as a single unit. This association gives them comfort when your young partner is caring for one of their patients.

They want assurance that you, as the senior partner and mentor, are lending a guiding hand in your partner's interaction with their patients, to ensure their safety and security. You should tell them this. Assure your referral base that you are a team and that together you, as a practice, will provide the most outstanding care for their patients.

It is important that you elevate the status of your partner in all interactions. First, I would avoid the use of the words "associate" and "junior." Introduce him as your partner. That not only makes him feel like an owner and gives him confidence, it also alleviates the anxiety of patients and referring physicians in a way that the other two terms do not. It does not diminish you in any way to elevate the status of your new partner. Quite the opposite.

Also, if you are truly trying to build a business, try to enhance your partner's reputation and encourage work to be sent his way. You must have the personal fortitude to watch proudly as your presumably younger partner begins to thrive and develop his own referral base. Sometimes this can be difficult for your own ego, but it is critical to the overall strategy of practice building.

A close friend of mine, who is a cardiologist, recently told me a story about being summoned into the office of a prominent cardiac surgeon. He said he felt like he was being called to the woodshed. He went to his office, and the surgeon sat him down and said to him, flat out, "Why are you sending so many patients to my junior partner? Why don't you send them to me? I sent you a couple of patients in recent weeks, because I wanted to remind you that I have a viable practice, too."

This demonstrated poor judgment on so many levels by this otherwise seasoned surgeon. First, he was creating tremendous discomfort in a physician who was a major referral source, if not directly to him, to his practice. Second, he diminished himself in the eyes of that physician. Third, he attempted to diminish his own partner in the eyes of what was already a major referrer.

Your strategy with a partner in your practice should be the exact opposite. Do everything that you can to use your own reputation to enhance the reputation of anyone associated with your practice. This will lead to faster, broader, and more sustained growth in both your partner's practice and your own. As his reputation grows, so does yours (by association), and, of course, as his business grows, so does yours.

Examine Your Insurance Strategy

I want to conclude this section with a brief discussion of a financial strategy that I have seen work countless times in practices with growing reputations and growing numbers of patients, partners, and revenues. Many physicians in large markets continue to be enrolled in any and all insurance plans that will have them on their panel. They do this regardless of the levels of reimbursement they provide, out of fear that they will be shut out. These doctors' real fear, of course, is that even their most steadfast referrers might hold back patients if they do not participate in every plan.

For a mature physician practice, I believe that it is worth re-evaluating this strategy. Using some of the tools from the previous section, "The Sharp Edge," you should be able to analyze each of your insurance plans to determine what your risk really is if you were to opt out of any individual plan.

Things to consider:
- volume and income from patients who come from these plans
- who the referrers are
- the impact on your valuable referral source if you choose to go out of network for the patients of one or another plan

Sometimes it pays to remain on a panel as a courtesy to a particularly important referral source. In some large cities, I know many physicians who have opted out of all insurance plans except Medicare. Even though Medicare is among the worst of the payers, these physicians continue to participate in order to keep their referrers happy.

You should be able to quite easily create a break-even analysis that shows how many patients you would need to keep in order to maintain the same level of income. I have been asked numerous times by friends and colleagues to help them perform such an analysis. They are frequently amazed at how much work they are doing for so little money for certain plans, and how unimportant it would be if all of that volume (and the small associated income) were to drop away.

An example: Years ago, when I did such an analysis of my own practice, I noticed that patients from one insurer made up 8 percent of my income and over 25 percent of my volume. As a result, I decided to opt out of the plan, willing to forgo this 8 percent of income. In a worst-case scenario, I figured none of those patients would stay with me if I dropped their plan.

But if I were to keep just one out of five of those patients, it would be a break-even for me financially, with more free time for additional cases. If I were to keep two patients, I would make a lot more money and be a little less busy—a home run, in my estimation. As it turned out, when I redid the analysis two years later, I found that I had kept four out of five patients—a grand slam!

I mention this here because expanding your practice to include a new partner makes such an analysis even more timely. If your reluctance to examine your ability to drop out of certain plans stems from your desire to capture all comers, or alternatively, from your fear of losing certain referrals, then you, as a practice, can create a mixed strategy where the more senior physician(s) can begin to eliminate some insurance plans with the understanding that the "junior partner(s)" will capture the spillover work.

In my experience with this strategy, only very rarely do patients leave the practice. More often than you would imagine, a patient will opt to go out of network for the so-called "name partner," thereby dramatically enhancing the practice's revenue. And only very rarely will the patient who is not willing to do this leave the practice entirely. Instead, the junior partner who does participate in the plan takes over his care. The referring physician should be reassured with the understanding that the senior physician will continue to lend guidance to the younger partner.

While becoming more selective about the insurance plans in which you participate frees you up for more lucrative work, this strategy has the additional benefit of helping to build volume and enhance the reputation of your younger partner. It also accelerates the time in which you can expand your practice even further, by adding additional partners. You can then employ the same strategy again and again in a cascading effect so that you build your reputation doing the work that is most meaningful to you, while ensuring you are fairly compensated.

Another important strategy to employ with your partner: Encourage and assist her in creating a referral base that is complementary to your own. For example, when contacting other physicians for consultations on your patients, encourage her to refer to physicians to whom you do not usually send patients.

By doing this, you are both likely to see new patients from referral sources that you had not previously enjoyed.

This is how practice empires are built.

Key Learning Points: How to Build a Practice

1. Nurturing relationships with referring physicians is perhaps the most important way to build your practice, as they hold the key to explosive growth. Understand their needs and exceed their expectations. Use key tools to communicate frequently.

2. Exceed your patients' expectations with respect to communication. Use tools, such as AIDET, printed practice information, and hand-drawn sketches.

3. Make post-visit phone calls. They reduce patient anxiety, complaints, and claims while improving clinical outcomes.

4. Remember to include family members in communication and be proactive and honest when communicating about complications.

5. Build your reputation by writing papers; speaking to community organizations, specialty societies, and those in your own organization; volunteering for leadership roles; and cultivating relationships with your staff, nurses, and residents.

6. Consider adding a junior partner. First run a financial analysis. Then use behavioral-based interview questions to ensure organizational fit. Manage up your new partner's reputation to patients and referral sources to build the practice.

7. Analyze your participation in various insurance plans. You may be able to opt out of plans that offer poor reimbursement while still retaining patient and referring physician loyalty.

CHAPTER 7

HOW TO DESTROY A PRACTICE IN 90 DAYS

· · · · · · · · · ·

As we have seen, building a practice and maintaining it is hard work. Unfortunately, destroying it is easy.

A little more than ten years ago, I had an idea. To this day, I still think it was an excellent idea, and at the time, so did the U.S. Patent Office, which, in fact, issued me a patent on its execution.

Basically, I was going to (and ultimately did) create a website that would serve as a focal point and resource for patients who had colostomies, ileostomies, and urostomies. The website would both provide information and allow purchases of certain appliances. The patent was issued for a specific technical aspect of this kind of commerce. In any event, I was certain that I was going to be an Internet mogul.

Around the same time, I was going through a period of disenchantment with my work...something that I believe every physician goes through at least once, if not multiple times, during the course of his or her career. I had somehow lost my mojo. I was no longer making the connection between what I was doing and the purpose and worthwhile nature of the work.

Over the next several months, I engaged in a number of activities that negatively impacted my practice.

Lesson #1: Be Hungry.

One of the maxims of success that is often quoted is, "Don't dress for the job you have. Dress for the job you want." Well, in 1999, I wanted to be an Internet mogul. And the uniform for players in the new, burgeoning online industry was shorts (torn blue jeans, if you had an important meeting), sandals, and old t-shirts. So for a while, I hung up my suits and dressed for the job I wanted.

I never really considered what this attire would make my patients think when I rounded on them in the hospital or saw them in my office. Imagine for yourself the difference between a guy in jeans and a sharply dressed clean-cut gentleman in a tie and a white coat. As a patient, I vote for the latter.

During those days, I did not ignore my patients, nor did I provide less than outstanding care, but instead of hanging out in the cafeteria and in the physician's lounge, or cruising through the emergency room (a strategy that I wholeheartedly endorse, particularly for younger physicians), I could often be found at my business partner's office 40 blocks away from the hospital. Or even better, I would go way downtown to Tribeca where the Web developers (mine and every other one on the planet) lived and worked.

With my referring physicians, I would always try to bring the conversation around to my new business and what I was creating. Again, I served my patients well and provided excellent care, but in looking back through the eyes of those referring physicians, I can only surmise that I failed to act like "an owner" or like I particularly cared about servicing their needs. In short, I lowered their barrier to exit from my practice.

This was particularly disruptive within my group. My practice volume dropped, my receipts plummeted, and my performance as a managing partner definitely took a big hit as a result.

My disengagement had a negative effect on the morale of our employees as well. I failed to make myself very available to manage their needs. At the end of the day, it cost me real money and had a profound effect on my practice.

But there were also many tremendous positives that came out of this experience. I did emerge from this period re-energized, re-engaged, and far more knowledgeable about the real nature of the business world. I tell this story to help illustrate some of the issues that can very rapidly cause serious damage to a previously highly functioning practice. Fortunately, I recovered, fairly quickly, and ultimately gained quite a bit more than I had lost.

Sometimes outside factors can do great damage, and it is important to recognize these and to mitigate the harm as quickly and as effectively as possible.

Another example: A colleague of mine had the good fortune (or ultimately, misfortune) of winning a fairly significant sum of money in the state lottery.

The amount he won could not have been worse. It was not nearly enough to make a huge difference in his life, and certainly not enough to allow for him to alter his practice or his lifestyle, but it was an amount that was high enough to make people think differently about him. Through no doing of his own, many people perceived him as no longer being "hungry," much the way I demonstrated myself to be during my Internet phase.

Many physicians stopped referring their patients to him and sent them instead to those they felt needed the work more. In the end, I believe my colleague lost much more than he won. Ultimately, he was able to again recover his practice, but I am not certain that he ever regained it at a level that matched its true potential.

I am an eternal optimist. I tend to accentuate the positive and downplay the negative. But in order to keep your edge, there are a few behaviors against which I feel the need to caution you in order to prevent the destruction of your practice. Here are some additional lessons I have learned.

Lesson #2: Do Not Disengage.

I'm always amused when patients thank me for returning their calls. When I ask them about it, they report that many doctors don't return their phone calls, either in a prompt manner or sometimes ever. Many of these patients end up asking me for referrals to other physicians when my limited intervention is completed.

Equally unacceptable is not returning phone calls from referring physicians. This is your lifeblood. I know a number of specialists who have reached a point where they will call several doctors simultaneously and give a case to whoever returns the call first. Because I established myself long ago as someone who always promptly returns calls, my referring doctors feel no need to employ this strategy. Make sure you can say the same thing.

Many doctors also disengage through nonverbal cues. This is something that patients, other doctors, and staff can sense easily, so be very aware of your body language. Relationship killers include things like standing instead of sitting down with a patient, looking at your watch, and—my favorite—answering phone calls or emails during a conversation. These are ultimately potential practice destroyers.

When I was a resident, I noticed that one doctor's patients always seemed to require more of my time on rounds than similar patients from another surgeon. His patients were more unsettled and required more explanation and handholding than those of his colleague. They often complained that the surgeon did not spend enough time with them, and that they felt that the explanations they were receiving were inadequate.

When I spoke to the other residents about it, we all concluded the same thing: This surgeon spent less time on rounds with his patients than the other surgeon did. Everything else was essentially equal. It was the same type of patient, the same demographic, and the same types of surgery by two highly skilled, excellent doctors, both of whom were personally charming and engaging. What else could we conclude?

So I did a study. I made rounds with both of them for several weeks. What I learned was enlightening. These two surgeons spent exactly the same amount of time with their patients. They had the same conversations. They spoke about the same things. They had the same combination of personal touch and engagement with their patients.

The only difference—and I mean the only one—was that one doctor sat down on the edge of the bed every time he saw a patient, while the other did not. And, in fact, the one who stood always seemed to be leaning towards the door. Even when he was having a conversation, even when he was not on his way out, his body language said, *I have somewhere else I need to be.*

Several studies have verified this. For example, a 2008 study at the Mayo Clinic College of Medicine[9] showed that when their doctors sat down, patients overestimated the time the doctors spent with them, whereas if the doctors stood, time spent was underestimated. Similarly, a 2005 study in another journal[10] found that patients whose physicians sat with them perceived their physicians to be more compassionate and willing to spend more time with them compared to other physicians. My personal experience confirms this.

As a busy surgeon from New York with an edge and a business mentality, I say to you, "Sit down every time you see a patient." It's good for business. It's also the right thing to do. It alleviates patient anxiety. It creates a bond. It makes the patient feel less vulnerable, and it makes him like you more. It makes him feel as if he were the only person you care about at that moment. Answering phone calls and emails—or leaning out the door—are behaviors that do not engender that feeling. And they are just plain rude.

Lesson #3: Do Not Disappear.

It is often said that a big part of life is just showing up. One way to rapidly lose your practice and the goodwill that you have built is to disappear.

How many of you have noticed that in the three days leading up to a vacation, you're the busiest doctor on the planet, but that as soon as you're back, even if you're gone for only a week, it's as if nobody ever heard of you? (In fact, I'm on vacation right now, and it's making me nervous as hell.)

As we discussed before in "How to Build a Practice," reminders of your availability are very effective tools at keeping your name in the forefront of the minds of your referring physicians. The converse is also true. From the perspective of a referring physician, you are easy to forget when those follow-up letters dry up or she doesn't bump into you in the hallway for several weeks. When she no longer sees you at breakfast in the cafeteria or gets your phone calls, it is just plain easier to refer patients to the doctor she did just get a note or call from. Unfortunately, it does not take long for referrals to dry up during your absence. I think it's just the nature of human beings to find new ways to meet their needs when the old ways are not as accessible or convenient. You must maintain your presence in your sphere of influence.

A particularly glaring example of this is when you stop attending department and hospital functions. This can include meetings, grand rounds, administrative functions, and even fundraisers or social events. While there are many important reasons to attend these events in the first place, an equally key reason is to keep patient referrals coming your way.

Another disappearing act that I believe is even more critical and more destructive to a practice is a failure to admit, apologize for, and most importantly, to manage complications of a patient's care.

Poor outcomes invariably happen. Early on, I was taught the maxim, "small surgery, small complications; big surgery, big complications." My assumption is that, like me, you are an excellent and committed physician—that you do everything in your power to prevent complications from occurring. But even in ideal circumstances, for example, anastomotic leaks from gastrointestinal anastomoses occur upwards of 2 to 3 percent of the time. And this is when conditions are ideal and the surgery is perfect.

So if you do 400 operations a year on the intestinal tract, which is not a huge number, then you can expect that about once a month you are likely to have a huge complication. And people are watching to see how you manage these patients and their families.

The surest way to engage in practice-destroying behavior is to become defensive or to be unsympathetic with the patients and their families and what they are going through. When you blame outside forces and events, or you fail to be present to care for your patient and his family, you let them down. You lose their trust and diminish your practice.

Frequently, I have watched an otherwise excellent physician disengage and disappear from the scene in such a situation due to either his fear of a lawsuit or his discomfort in dealing openly with the family and referring physician. This is exactly the wrong course to take.

Proper management of a complication requires increasing time spent with the patient and his family, stepping up communication, setting aside defensive posturing, demonstrating empathy, and, when appropriate, making an apology.

Failure to use these behaviors is extremely disruptive to building a practice, and, as has been shown time and again, is far more likely to result in litigation. This then tends to lead to a cycle of even greater disengagement and disappearance that can destroy your practice.

Lesson #4: Do Not Disown.

Another potential way to destroy a practice is to buy someone else's practice or sell your own to a third party. Increasingly, in this era of declining reimbursement and higher expectations and costs, physician practices are becoming owned by third parties, which are frequently hospitals or large multi-specialty groups. (In fact, according to the American Medical Association[11], in 2008, 77.4 percent of physicians practiced in group practice and/or hospital settings. This number continues to rise.)

One of the problems with this trend is that while hospitals are typically run by astute hospital managers, they do not necessarily have the skill set required to run individual physician practices. In fact, we are seeing a resurgence of a trend that occurred in the early years of the HMO onslaught. During the early 1990s, hospitals and large groups bought up physician practices in order to capture the capitated business of the HMOs. Unfortunately, many of these arrangements were doomed from the start.

More recently, it has been suggested that both RVU and receipt productivity of recently acquired practices is demonstrably decreased when measured against the same practices immediately prior to sale. This is not to say that only physicians owning private practices are able to retain their edge. Physician employees of large groups or members of university faculty practices are among the most productive physicians anywhere. It is when practices are bought out for more than their intrinsic values (adding so-called "goodwill" payments), and the retained physicians are then compensated without regard to continued productivity, that issues can arise.

Perhaps physicians feel that they can rest on their laurels when they sell their practices to larger groups and/or hospitals and become employees. There is a danger in adopting a "renter" mentality when moving from an ownership position to employee. Failure to maintain a sense of ownership and control is often the death knell for a successful clinical practice.

Interestingly, the colleague I spoke of earlier—the one who had complained about his call center—was just such a doctor. Several years ago, he had been in a highly successful private practice and had recently become hospital-employed. His is a perfect example of the change in mentality that can occur.

Lesson #5: Do Not "Dis."

We're all guilty of "dissing" others. At some point, in order to attempt to make ourselves look and possibly feel better, we have engaged in conversation that includes disparaging others, employing a potentially destructive strategy best described as "managing down."

We do it all the time. When a patient complains about waiting forever, you say that the transporters are slow and are to blame. You wholeheartedly nod agreement when your colleagues complain about radiology services. You confirm your patients' complaints that the nurses are short-staffed. You agree that the residents aren't as good as when you were a resident. The cafeteria stinks. The place is old and dingy. The OR schedule is a disaster. This patient is a jerk.

His family is too demanding. And, my favorite: The other specialist you saw for a second opinion is an idiot—I'm amazed that he got his license back!

I could go on all day. In fact, it is actually quite easy to manage people down, and it makes some people feel better about themselves. At least in the moment. But it is tremendously destructive, not only to the people and departments and institutions that you are disparaging, but also, ultimately, to yourself and your own practice.

> **Managing others *down*, rather than managing them *up*, also creates a "we/they" mentality between you and your patients, you and your staff, you and the hospital, and so on.**

This makes it very difficult to align goals, expectations, and outcomes. In the end, it makes your job harder. More importantly, it reflects poorly on *you*.

Try this: The next time your patient tells you that she saw one of your competitors in consultation prior to seeing you, instead of trying to find a clever way to close the deal with this patient, go the other way and see what happens. Instead of saying, "Yeah, he's a young guy. I helped train him. I imagine he's done one or two of these procedures as opposed to the hundreds that I've done," say something like, "Oh, he's excellent. I'm glad that you saw him as well. You're in great hands either way. You just have to do whatever makes you feel most comfortable."

I guarantee you that nine times out of ten, you will be the one caring for that patient. And in the tenth case, the patient will report back to your competitor that you said such nice things about him. Additionally, that patient will feel better about the decision that she made, and you will have done the right thing by alleviating her anxiety instead of adding to it.

Think about the employees you have hired. When was the last time you hired an employee who said that the reason she left her old job was that her boss was an idiot? My guess is never. According to Gallup, the number one reason employees leave their jobs is their supervisor. But a smart prospective employee never manages down her prior employer in a job interview. It would diminish her and make you wonder what she will soon be saying about you. For the same reason, managing down in any environment is never recommended.

Key Learning Points: How to Destroy a Practice 90 Days

1. Be hungry.

2. Do not disengage.

3. Do not disappear.

4. Do not disown.

5. Do not "dis."

CHAPTER 8

GROWING LOYALTY

· · · · · · · · · · ·

My current chairman, boss, and longtime mentor loves to spend time coaching me on leadership. He sums up his management style in terms of trying to be of service to those who work with him. He takes great pride in his ability to foster loyalty in those around him. And this has served him well.

I have watched him over the past 25 years as he grew from resident to fellow, became an entrepreneur, an attending, division chief, and now chairman, and it is hard to argue with the success of his approach. He is surrounded by people who have served him and the enterprise loyally for years, who understand and anticipate his needs, and who are comfortable and confident enough in their positions to take risks and challenge business as usual. In this chapter, we will discuss some specific tools and techniques that you can use to engender loyalty among your staff, colleagues, and patients.

Create a No-Tolerance Culture for Disruptive Behavior

I take great pride in the fact that people seem to enjoy working with me. My employee turnover is close to zero. The few times that my employees have left were when their career growth brought new opportunities. When such an event occurs, I celebrate their success rather than feel regret at my loss.

There are a number of things that you can do to help create an environment where your employees are tremendously loyal to you and your organization, and almost none of them have to do with money. Yes, you need to pay people in the range that is appropriate for their level of education, skill, and effort. But as I mentioned in Chapter 7, it is well documented that the primary reason employees leave their jobs is due to their relationships with their managers.

This is particularly true for physicians and their relationships with those who support them. In far too many cases, physicians are short, rude, or outright disrespectful to staff. Just recently, a fellow physician leader told me of a specialist in his department who yelled at and intimidated an excellent medical assistant who had been with them for 12 years.

As she exited a patient room, this physician confronted her in a public hallway. He aggressively approached her and yelled, "So when am I supposed to get the things in the room to do the biopsy?" She responded that she had not been informed that he needed these instruments, but her co-worker was standing just behind him with all instruments in hand. He continued to glare at her as she squeezed past him in the hallway.

She described the encounter as humiliating and disrespectful and felt embarrassed to be treated in such a way in front of her colleagues. His lack of professional courtesy reduced her to tears. And as she so aptly noted, "No matter what title a person has, he should never feel it's acceptable to act in a way that belittles someone else."

Research shows that nearly three in four healthcare providers have experienced some type of disruptive or intimidating behavior in the course of their work. And here's why that is just plain dangerous: Disruptive behavior leads to poor communication. How likely do you think this medical assistant will be to speak up in the future if she needs to inform this intimidating physician about a patient issue or medical error? Not very. Poor communication leads to gaps in quality and safety and creates risk for poor clinical outcomes.

When physicians don't hold themselves to the same standards of behavior they ask of their staff, it leads to employee dissatisfaction. In fact, in a study by Studer Group and Vanderbilt University Medical Center in Nashville, 66 percent of surveyed healthcare workers stated that they have considered leaving their jobs as a result of disruptive behavior by physicians.[12]

Celebrate Your Staff

In a medical practice, your staff perform a variety of *critical* functions. Respect their work. Never diminish what they do. You cannot provide the excellent care you do if your phones are not answered appropriately and the paperwork is not completed properly. If your scheduling is not efficient, you will pay the price. If patients are not greeted warmly and cared for with respect and compassion, your ability to have a meaningful clinical encounter may be compromised. And, as you remember from Chapter 2, the diligence and skill with which billing and collections are performed will have a great bearing on your personal profitability.

I admit it. I can't do their jobs. I have neither the mindset nor the skill set. And realistically, I don't have the patience to do some of the things that my staff does. As a result, I let them know at every opportunity how much I respect and appreciate what they do for me and for our patients.

CONNECT BACK TO PURPOSE.

> **It is important to remind your staff not only of the respect you have for the work that they do, but also to always connect the dots between what they do every day and how it makes a difference in the lives of your patients. Remind them frequently that you are a team with complementary skill sets that is engaged in the care of patients and their families.**

There is a great story that appears in Kevin and Jackie Freiberg's book *Guts! Companies That Blow the Doors Off Business-as-Usual* about a reporter's interview with Michael DeBakey, the famous heart surgeon. It is said that as he was walking down the hall during the interview, he encountered an elderly janitor who was mopping the floors of the hospital in which he worked.

Dr. DeBakey stopped and thanked the janitor. He reminded the janitor that what he was doing was important to patient care. He told the janitor that by cleaning the floors, he was creating an environment of patient safety. That he was, by his work, lowering the chances that the patients having heart surgery would get infections and potentially serious complications as a result.

It is said that later the reporter circled back and asked the janitor exactly what his function was in the hospital. And the janitor is said to have replied, "Me and Dr. DeBakey, we save lives together." My advice: Strive to be like Dr. DeBakey when you interact with your staff.

EDUCATE YOUR STAFF.

Be a teacher. Teach them about your business and share your clinical expertise. Your staff are interested in what you do and enjoy learning about the practice of medicine. It is good to remember from time to time that not everybody has gone to medical school.

Because you are surrounded daily by other physicians who have remarkably similar experiences, it can be easy to forget that you are part of a relatively small and privileged group of people who have the honor, training, and education to care for those who are ill and their families. It is important to remember that many of your staff got into healthcare for the same reasons. They care.

By sharing with your staff what you do and teaching them about your specialty, you re-ignite the spark of their own desire to make a difference in the lives of others. When you explain to them the reasons for the things that you do with your patients, they remember why they went into this field in the first place, and they become more effective. As they connect more authentically with you, your patients, and your referring physicians, they will feel greater satisfaction serving alongside you on a daily basis.

REWARD AND RECOGNIZE.

What a wonderful feeling it is as a physician when a patient tells you about the positive impact you have had on his or her life. How arrogant it would be to think that you alone are responsible for making such a difference. Share this praise with your staff. Let them know when patients express gratitude to you or gush about how great your office is. Pass on compliments from your happy large referrers about the seamless way in which phone calls and paperwork are handled. It costs nothing and the ROI is enormous.

I recognize that many of you are not necessarily the direct supervisors of your staff. But even if you are the junior partner in a group practice or one of many physicians in a large multi-specialty group or academic environment, this still holds true. Even if you are not in a position to hire, fire, or directly evaluate employees, you can make a point of complimenting a job well done or step up to provide teaching opportunities.

BE AN ADVOCATE.

If you want your staff to be loyal, you must be loyal to them. Speak up for the people with whom you work. Advocate for them with management to ensure they have the tools and equipment they need to do their jobs. It might be as simple as requesting that the fax machine be moved into a position that is more ergonomically satisfying to your secretary, or as complicated as pushing for education or additional training for those of your staff who you think have the potential to grow. Even if your input is not solicited, you can demonstrate the kind of leadership that enhances and promotes your staff.

COMMUNICATE.

Communication is critical to ensure day-to-day workflow and patient outcomes, so meet frequently with each member of your team, whether in groups or individually. These meetings should have three distinct and clear functions: rounding, strategic planning, and mentoring.

First, just as we round with our colleagues to ensure that our patients' needs are met in the hospital, rounding with individual staff members can be an extremely effective tool in the outpatient environment.

Each week, after my office hours, I meet with my medical assistant to go over patients not only from that day but for the entire month. In 15 minutes, we are able to go over the status of everyone we have seen together—patient by patient—for the prior four weeks. This way we don't miss anything, we are aligned in our approach going forward, and we ensure that the care plan for every patient we have seen is clear.

By reviewing cases from a month earlier, we are able to review the outcomes of any tests or consultations and create and document a follow-up plan. This ensures that nothing falls through the cracks. We also generate a list of follow-up phone calls that I will make to patients. My medical assistant becomes an integral part of creating this superior level of care and service to our patients.

The second type of meeting I recommend you hold with members of your team is for the purpose of practice strategy. To think that you alone—or even management alone or the group of physicians alone—have the answers to on-going strategic planning is a bit arrogant. Create an environment of transparency and information in your practice by including your staff in strategic planning. It builds loyalty and engagement to both you and the enterprise.

The third kind of meeting, which should always be performed on a one-to-one basis, is for the purpose of mentorship. You are a leader. Whether you realize it or not, you are also a mentor. You can use this position to further strengthen your relationship with your employees by understanding and helping them achieve the goals that they set for themselves in their careers. They want your guidance.

Ultimately, as I stated earlier, you will lose some of these people as they move on to bigger and better things. And while this may seem disruptive to your practice, it really is far less of a burden than holding back someone who has the potential and the desire to expand her horizons. Additionally, she will be an ambassador for you throughout the remainder of her career. Think for a moment about the university from which you graduated, and its pride in populating the world with its graduates in a variety of different fields. In a small way, this is what you are accomplishing when you mentor your own employees.

FIRE LOW PERFORMERS.

If you have an employee with whom no one else seems to be able to work, take early action. When high performers are forced to work with low performers, they get the message that you do not value high performance. As a result, they will pace themselves, look for a job elsewhere, or put their energies into something besides work to find satisfaction. One low performer puts your entire staff at risk. (For tips and strategies on how to manage high-, middle-, and low-performing employees, search on "highmiddlelow" at StuderGroup.com.)

Additionally, you may find that, despite practicing all of the techniques described above, one or more of your employees still don't seem to get it. They don't respond to your teaching efforts. They don't quite become an integral part of your team. This, too, warrants a search for a replacement. There are enough good people who are looking for worthwhile work and the ability to make a difference that you should not need to settle for less.

Earn Loyalty from Colleagues and Referrers

In Chapter 5, we discussed the concept of relationship marketing and creating a barrier to exit. This concept is essentially synonymous with loyalty. Your ultimate goal is to create an environment with your referrers where it would be difficult for them to call anyone other than you to service those needs in which you have a particular expertise. Taking that thought a step further, I would say it is even better if your colleagues call you for things that are not in your area of expertise, and you manage those as well.

In my case, I don't do vascular surgery. I don't manage epidural catheters. I don't put in chest tubes for pneumothoraces. And I don't do orthopedic surgery. But I'm sure glad when I get a call from one of my referring physicians who asks me to manage one of these problems.

And how do you think I respond?

Do you think I say, "Oh, no, I don't manage that"?

Of course not. I say, "Don't worry. I'll take care of it." It's the mature practitioner's version of what I shared with you earlier from my days as a resident: "Done. What else?"

Of course, do not practice out of your field. Help identify the best person to manage a particular problem. In this setting, you are doing a service for your referrer and his patient, but not necessarily directly providing care.

The best way to maintain the loyalty of your colleagues and referrers is to take care of them and their problems immediately, effectively, and completely. Essentially, give them the same kind of care you would give a patient.

Be their instrument. First, check your ego at the door. Then make happen for them and their patients whatever needs to be done, whether it is in your field or not...whether you are going to get praise, credit, money, or not. And in the process, manage them up.

How do you think my friend, the gastroenterologist, feels when his patient returns to him and says, "Dr. Harris thinks you're the greatest thing since sliced bread. He told me that you know more about Crohn's Disease than Crohn himself." Do you think he's angry? Do you think he feels silly or embarrassed? No. He feels wonderful on many levels.

First, he knows that the patient sitting in front of him feels that she is lucky to be there at that moment, with this gastroenterologist. He knows that she feels that she is getting the best care, both with him and with me. And he knows that the next time, or the next ten times, that he refers a patient to me, he is going to get a similar response. Everybody wins, including the patient.

Another thing to keep in mind, as you care for your referring physicians and their patients, is that they, too, have staff. And their staff have the same issues as yours do. They, too, want to be reminded of their role and their importance in patient care. Treat them as if they were the referring physicians.

Demonstrate the respect that you have for their work. This does not undermine their own employers. Quite the opposite. It reinforces that their mentors have selected appropriately by choosing you to help them, the staff, care for "their" patients.

When I call a doctor's office, I make the call myself. I never have my staff do it. And I never say I'm Doctor Harris. When I call a physician, whether it is one I know or one I don't, I introduce myself as Mickey Harris. The ones who know me know I'm a doctor. And the ones who don't figure it out fairly quickly. But I have already established a bond with the staff that suggests that I do not hold myself in a superior position to them...that I respect them and the work that they do in helping me to care for their patients. The other thing that I am accomplishing by doing this, by making the calls myself, is that I am respecting their time.

How often has *this* happened: Your administrative assistant calls you on the intercom and says, "Dr. Friedman is calling." You pick up the phone and say, "Bob?" And the voice responds, "No. This is Sonya from Dr. Friedman's office. Let me get Dr. Friedman for you."

When I call a physician, I never summon him or her to wait for me. To me, that demonstrates a lack of respect, and it certainly does not engender loyalty.

Care for Your Patients

When you manage your patients, create an environment of comfort and caring. This creates a valuable patient/physician bond, which engenders loyalty in many ways. To learn many excellent techniques for exceeding your patients' expectations, I refer you to Dr. Beeson's book *Practicing Excellence*. It is a wonderful instruction manual on how to deliver exceptional healthcare. I will share a few thoughts here, however, with respect to engendering patient loyalty to you and your practice.

First, be great. While I have already said that being clinically great is not enough, and that quality is not a point of differentiation between you and your competitors, it is, indeed, the absolute minimum. At the very least, start there. Be great.

Next, remember why the patients are there. Patients are not sitting across from you to torture you, to bother you, to prevent you from being with your family. They are there because they are having major life events. The better you can remember that, and the more that you can express your empathy with them, the more loyalty you will create.

> **Doctors and nurses often share with me that they're having a difficult day. They're tired. They're angry. They're bored. They're miserable. My response to them is always the same. I tell them that whenever I think I'm having a bad day, I remember that my very worst day is better than the day that my patient is having.**

I truly believe that if you say this to yourself, if you remind yourself of this, in those words, you will never have a bad day practicing medicine again.

Remember that your patients' families are having a rough time, too. Patients are not alone in their journeys. Most patients have families, friends, or loved ones who accompany them and who are suffering alongside them. They, too, are looking to you for comfort. And in my experience, patients, as sick as they may be, are remarkably selfless. They are as concerned with the welfare of their loved ones as they are with their own issues.

Part of the measure of you as a physician is how you care for the family members of your patients. So my advice to you, with respect to creating loyal patients, is to care for their families as if they were, themselves, the patients. Acknowledge them. Learn their names. Engage them in conversation. And let them know that you are cognizant of and respect their feelings and their desires for their loved ones to receive the best possible care for their illnesses. Not only will they respond, but the patient will feel a tremendous comfort and yes, loyalty, to you for including them, as she has, in her care.

I received a note the other day from a patient, reproduced in the figure below.

Dear Dr. Harris,

I wanted to drop you a quick note to thank you for meeting with my brother, Steven, and me. I appreciate all the time you spent with us, and you made us feel like we were the only people you had as patients. You have a very caring nature as well as being very warm and personable. I am most grateful Dr. Itzkowitz sent me to you. I feel I am in "good hands." Of course, I am anxious and a wee bit nervous, yet I know I will be well and that is my focus.

So, I will see you soon. Thank you again for being so concerned with my well-being and making me feel comfortable with what is going to happen.

Warm regards,
Lesleigh Strauss

As you can see, she remarks that they felt that they were the only thing that mattered to me at that moment, that they were the only patient and family I was caring for. They knew fully well that I was busy. They knew that I had a packed schedule in my office that day, and that later she was one of many patients I was visiting in the hospital on my rounds after surgery. And yet, at any given moment, they did not feel as such. In fact, soon after Ms. Strauss's surgery, I also received a beautiful note from her brother, thanking me for how I treated *him*, as well as his sister.

In the same vein, allow your patients to see how you treat your staff, your colleagues, and your other patients. We have already discussed how managing others down diminishes you in the eyes of those to whom you do this. The converse holds equally true. The more generous you are with your praise, the more comfortable you are in deflecting kudos towards your supporting staff, the more humble you are about your own skill and contribution to the patient's care, the more she elevates you in her own mind and feels that she is in caring and generous hands.

I also remember that I got a phone call while I was making rounds on her second postoperative day. My hip buzzed, and then it began to ring. I didn't take the call. Instead, I very clearly stated, "I'm sorry, but this can wait. Let me turn this off so that we're not interrupted again."

Remember the book *The House of God*? I hope you have read it at least four or five times. In this book, and then subsequently through my residency, even at a Level 1 trauma center, I learned that there was no emergency so great that it required running.

> **By the same token, there is nothing that can't wait until you have finished a conversation with your patient. We have all become too reliant on instant communication, and urgency has given way to rudeness.**

As important as respecting your time with patients is the need to respect your patients' time. All too often, we show patients and their families that we think more highly of our own time than theirs. Nowhere is that more evident than in the office setting where physicians routinely keep patients waiting for minutes if not hours on end. I think it is safe to say that each of us believes our time to be important.

Unfortunately, most of us, as physicians, stop there. And this is a major source of dissatisfaction for our patients.

The way to obtain the loyalty of your patients is to take the next step by demonstrating to them, "I recognize and respect the fact that your time is as important to you as my time is to me."

So be on time. One way to demonstrate respect for patients is to be on time in our office hours. The idea that patients are willing to wait for "better" caregivers is, at best, archaic. If you, as a physician, can manage your office hours so that you are programmed to be on time, that would go a long way towards creating loyalty among your patients. If you cannot be on time, apologize. And be sincere. Tell the patient that you respect his time, and that you will make it worth his wait.

Along these lines, I believe that improving access is a goal that is worthy of enormous thought and resources in our current system. One way that we have addressed the ability to improve access and respect patients' time is through the use of scheduling templates. I refer you to our website, FireStarterPublishing.com/ExcellenceWithAnEdge, for examples of their use.

In one of our practices, we improved overall patient satisfaction from the 3rd percentile to the 35th percentile within a matter of weeks, merely by utilizing such templates for patient scheduling.

Make Mistakes, But Own Up to Them

I make mistakes. I'd bet you make mistakes, too. Most people do. Since organizations are run by people, it follows, then, that even the best-run organizations make mistakes. A big difference between good and great organizations is how they respond when the inevitable lapse in service occurs. In business parlance, this is called "service recovery."

We have previously discussed how best to manage poor medical outcomes. Here, I am referring to things like scheduling errors, cancellations, delays, and billing errors...all of the annoying things that occur in your practice, and in all industries, whether avoidable or not. How well you manage these occurrences will to a great extent determine the loyalty of your patients and referrers.

I once stayed at a Ritz-Carlton, and it was great. Until I got the bill. I had made a few brief phone calls to my kids less than 20 miles away (though in another area code), and saw a charge of almost $75 added to my bill.

I went to the front desk prepared for a fight, fully expecting to have to ask for a manager. But after a discussion with the desk clerk, she said, "I'm really sorry about this. I will remove it from your bill. I hope that everything else about your stay with us was to your liking."

By resolving my complaint immediately during our first encounter, they gained a loyal customer. (I later learned that all Ritz-Carlton employees are empowered to spend up to $2,000 a day to resolve customer complaints. In *USA Today*[13], Vice President Diana Oreck said hotel standards are so high and service-recovery training is so rigorous that no employee has ever had to provide a $2,000 credit.)

This story demonstrates an important tenet of customer service, which is that customers who have a problem and don't complain, don't return. Customers who have a problem, and do complain, have a much higher retention rate, especially if their problem is resolved by the first person they encounter. Retention rates fall dramatically if complaints are poorly or slowly managed.[14]

We can also apply this principle to medical practice. While I am by no means suggesting that you give your receptionist carte blanche to give thousands of dollars away to your patients just because you are a few minutes late, I am suggesting that you will build and maintain patient loyalty by recognizing that people respond well to sincere apologies and swift complaint resolution. Likewise, they will tend to leave your practice when ignored or rebuffed.

The How-tos of Service Recovery

First, train your front desk staff to anticipate and respond to complaints. Merely saying, "I'll talk to the doctor," or, "I'll tell the manager," more often inflames rather than soothes the anger of patients and their families. Saying the words, "I'm sorry," will go a very long way with a patient, unless it is immediately followed by, "but it's not my fault."

Give your staff specific scripts for handling situations that you know will come up periodically...like when you are delayed due to an emergency. Empower them to rectify problems without needing to call someone else.

Possible solutions include: rescheduling appointments with the promise of being taken immediately at the rescheduled time, having the patient seen by your partner, buying the patient and/or family members a cup of coffee, or paying for parking. I know one practice that has ordered a catered lunch for patients and their families who have had to wait to see the doctor. One critical thing to remember here, though, is that you must deliver on the promised remedy, or you will never see that patient, or anyone he or she knows, again.

For larger groups, it may prove worthwhile to have a specific person or program dedicated to service recovery. In my department, we have created a position called the "patient advocate," whose main function is to serve as a focus for service recovery. She spends much of her time interacting with patients in the reception areas of our practices, dealing with delays and other lapses in service before they escalate into difficult problems.

The patient advocate has special training in how to deal effectively with angry patients and their families, and is available to be called in by our front desk staff whenever patient complaints exceed the commonly scripted issues with which they typically deal. She will alleviate the problem and always follows up with a call and/or letter to the patient in order to complete the recovery.

Our physicians, patients, and staff have found the patient advocate to be an invaluable resource, and our patient satisfaction survey results reflect this. In fact, in the last several months, at least three other departments in our faculty practice have created similar positions modeled on ours.

While seemingly a potentially expensive endeavor, spending on customer service and, in particular, service recovery, has been shown across all industries to be a worthwhile investment. Remember that just as the cost of recruiting new staff far exceeds the cost of retaining loyal employees, the same holds true of customers (patients and referring physicians) as well.

Additional Thoughts on Growing Loyalty

As you can see, creating and maintaining loyalty from staff, colleagues, and patients falls into just a few broad categories of interpersonal interaction. First, as Studer Group recommends, "Manage up!" This not only elevates those around you, it also elevates your stature in the eyes of your staff, colleagues, and patients.

Next, always do the right thing. Whenever faced with a choice of expedience or moral correctness, choose the latter. Be a mensch! Always.

Also, frequently remind yourself and the people around you of what it is that you are working towards together. Connect people back to their sense of purpose and worthwhile work. Show them how the work that they do and the effort that they make directly results in better outcomes for your patients. This is noble work. Say so often.

And finally, remember that you are a leader. Whether you are the CEO of a huge multi-specialty group or hospital, or you are a first-year, employed physician just out of residency, you have the ability and the stature to guide the people around you, so please do so.

Keep this in mind and loyalty will follow. And so will success. It has to.

Key Learning Points: Growing Loyalty

1. Celebrate and nurture your staff. Teach them about your specialty, reward and recognize them with compliments, and communicate consistently.

2. Create a no-tolerance culture for disruptive behavior. Disruptive behaviors lead to poor communication with staff, which puts patient safety at risk.

3. Retain high performers by removing low performers.

4. Earn loyalty from colleagues and referrers. Take care of their problems immediately, effectively, and completely. Treat them the way you would treat a patient.

5. Care for your patients. Create an environment of comfort and caring for patients and their families. Be respectful of their time.

6. Focus on service recovery.

7. Be a mensch. Always do the right thing.

SECTION 3
WHAT EXCELLENCE WITH AN
edge
LOOKS LIKE

So far, we have examined a variety of concepts and principles, and have reviewed many specific tools that you can utilize to provide better patient care, grow your practice and reputation, promote loyalty among your patients, referring physicians, and staff, and optimize your financial performance.

In this section, we will follow the course of a single patient encounter through three sets of eyes—those of the referring physician, the staff, and the patient. This is what excellence with an edge looks like.

I would love to be able to say that this is the way it happens with every patient in my practice every time. Unfortunately, I can't. The encounter described in the next pages is an idealized version of practice that represents the standard I continually strive to meet. As humans working with other humans, we are, of course, imperfect. But my goal is to hardwire a culture of *always*. Every patient every time.

CHAPTER 9

THE REFERRING PHYSICIAN EXPERIENCE

· · · · · · · · · ·

When Dr. Stevens sees a patient with Crohn's disease who may require an ileo-colic resection, he already knows that I'm his guy. I have established with him a track record of easy communication, outstanding patient care, and superior service. It is easy for him to recommend me.

Pre-Referral

Dr. Stevens knows that if there is a complex problem about which he needs to speak with me, he has my cell phone number and my back line as well. He knows that my staff has been instructed to expedite our communication and to respond to his needs. And he knows that his patient will come back to him happy and well, and that he, Dr. Stevens, will enjoy an enhanced reputation.

Referral

When Dr. Stevens gives Mrs. Miller my name and office number, he may manage me up by explaining that I operated on his mother. He may tell the patient that she is going to get great care, because we often make rounds together in the hospital, and, philosophically, we are always on the same page. He's not worried about the patient's cardiac disease, because he knows that once the phone call is made, I will make sure that it is managed.

In this case, he gives Mrs. Miller my office number and tells her to make an appointment to see me as soon as possible. He knows that I'll be able to see her within a few days or a week at the very outside. If he needs me to see the patient today, he will call me directly.

Pre-Visit

Two days before the patient is scheduled to see me, Dr. Stevens has already moved on from this referral to focus on his other patients. However, he gets a phone call from me while his staff hands him Mrs. Miller's chart. His staff has already sent copies of all of his important notes, test results, and correspondence at the request of my medical assistant. I remind him that I am about to consult on a patient of his. The first thing I do is thank him for the referral. I tell him that I have reviewed his notes and the films and get right to the point. I ask him for his thoughts and let him know that I'll get back to him as soon as I have seen the patient.

Post-Visit

Two days later, I call Dr. Stevens again. I review my findings briefly and let him know my thoughts. Together we agree on a plan of action. I also tell Dr. Stevens that during my consultation with Mrs. Miller, I learned that her mother had suffered from some kind of bleeding disorder that had never been worked up.

To be thorough and safe, I explain that I believe a pre-operative hematology consultation is indicated in this setting. I ask Dr. Stevens which hematologist he would like the patient to see. I also ask him if he wants to make that phone call, or if he prefers that I do it. He knows that if I call, I'm going to be sure that the hematologist knows that this is a consult from Dr. Stevens rather than from me. I thank him again for allowing me to assist in his patient's care. I use those words.

Pre-Op

Several days later, Dr. Stevens receives a letter from me. The first thing the letter contains is a "thank-you." It goes on to explain that I have enclosed the detailed consultation note from my electronic medical record. The cover letter is on heavy bond stationery, with my letterhead, and briefly outlines the highlights of our plan. Once again, the closing of the letter includes another thank-you for including me in his patient's care. (To view an example of such a letter, visit FireStarterPublishing.com/ExcellenceWithAnEdge.)

In the meantime, our offices have been in communication. Dr. Stevens' office staff knows the time and date that the patient will be operated upon and has been asked to put this on Dr. Stevens' calendar. By this time, Mrs. Miller has probably already circled back with Dr. Stevens by phone, at my request, to close the loop and assure the patient that we are all on the same page. Both Dr. Stevens and the patient are comforted by this exchange.

Peri-Op

As soon as I am done with Mrs. Miller's surgery, I call Dr. Stevens. I do this even before going to see the patient's family to let them know that she is out of surgery and doing well. I tell Dr. Stevens exactly what was done during the operation and alert him to any specific issues or concerns. I also, of course, share the specific details of any intra-operative complications that may have occurred.

I tell Dr. Stevens that I am now going to see Mrs. Miller's family and that I will make sure to tell them that we have spoken. I also tell him that I will pass on his good wishes to them. When I do go see the family, I do just that. I let them know that I have already spoken with Dr. Stevens and that he wishes their loved one well. The family is comforted, and Dr. Stevens is elevated in the esteem of the family.

Hospital Course

Dr. Stevens or one of his partners will likely round daily on this patient. In a routine recovery, I make sure that I see the patient early every day and that I write clear, legible, timed notes in the patient's record that accurately and specifically communicate to Dr. Stevens what is happening and what I am thinking. If anything—and I mean anything—out of the routine occurs, he will get a phone call from me. I also make sure that it is clear that the cardiac issues have been attended to and are continuing to be monitored. On the day of discharge, I make sure that Dr. Stevens knows the discharge plan and that his input is included. I also ensure that his request for follow-up has been correctly relayed to the patient.

In the case of a referring physician who is not on staff at my hospital, I will ask the doctor at the time of the surgery how often he would like me to call. I make sure that I call at least once every two to three days, even when things are going well and, of course, the second there is a problem. I also call him upon the patient's discharge. Dr. Stevens should never get a phone call from a family member asking about a problem that I have not already reported to him.

Follow-Up

Every patient receives a call from me within 48 hours after discharge from the hospital. If any issues are brought to light during that conversation, I will call Dr. Stevens to keep him informed. Often, if this was a very complicated case, I will call Dr. Stevens anyway just to let him know that the patient has been home for a couple of days and is doing quite well.

Almost all patients come back to see me approximately two weeks following their discharge. Barring a problem (which, of course, warrants a phone call), Dr. Stevens will receive a letter from me detailing the progress of the patient noted at that visit. Attached will be the official operative report and pathology report for his records. In the closing of the letter, I will make it clear whether or not I will need to see the patient again or if I am discharging her back to his complete care.

The patient will follow up with a visit to Dr. Stevens, whose chart is up-to-date with clear and complete information about all that has transpired. And, I am certain, the patient will thank Dr. Stevens as if he himself had performed the surgery.

CHAPTER 10

THE STAFF EXPERIENCE

· · · · · · · · · · ·

Pre-Referral

Before Mrs. Miller even calls my office, my staff are ready. They have been with me for an average of seven years. They were initially selected following a set of interviews during which specific behavioral questions were asked and discussed. We all share a sense of purpose, worthwhile work, and making a difference.

In addition to the standard training they have received from our medical center, each of my staff has also spent a great deal of time with me throughout his or her tenure, to ensure that we are always on the same page in caring for and providing the best possible service to our patients and families.

On each of their desks is the Team Harris Credo, which they themselves created:

> Our team's mission is to exceed the expectations of our patients, their families, their referring doctors, and, whenever possible, our colleagues and co-workers.

They each have been to the operating room with me on at least one occasion, and have seen firsthand the nature of the surgery that we do, as well as the experience that our patients undergo when we provide surgical care. Through seminars, I have reinforced their knowledge of the services that we provide.

And they have been given scripts so they know how to negotiate a variety of different scenarios to ensure we project ourselves consistently to our patients, their families, and referring physicians.

Referral

When Mrs. Miller calls, the phone is answered. By a live human. Most of the time, it will be my medical assistant, but if not, one of my other employees—who is fully aware that at this moment it is her responsibility, and is fully trained to do so—will answer the phone. And she will say, every time, "Good morning, Surgical Associates. This is Sarah. How may I help you?"

When Mrs. Miller tells her that she was given my name by Dr. Stevens, Sarah will manage up both Dr. Stevens and me. She will find something true to tell the patient—something along the lines of, "Oh, Dr. Stevens is terrific, isn't he? Dr. Harris and Dr. Stevens work together all the time."

When making the consultation appointment with Mrs. Miller, Sarah will determine the general reason for the visit. She will then offer an appointment time based on a template that has been created in our scheduling system. This template was created and is periodically updated in order to ensure ideal patient flow during the office day. Its use makes both the scheduling and the actual appointment go more smoothly.

Sarah will spend a considerable amount of time on this phone call, both obtaining and imparting information, all the while using her AIDET skills to alleviate any anxiety that the patient may have. She will arrange to get all of the records from Dr. Stevens' office and any that the patient may have in her possession. She will give by phone, by email, by fax, and/or by U.S. mail a whole host of information about me, our practice, and the logistics of how we work. She will remind the patient that by completing and returning requested information in a timely manner, the patient will optimize her visit in my office.

Included in this packet is information about parking, public transportation, the building, the hospital, and billing. Also included is an "intake form" on which the patient can easily write her medical history so that I can review it prior to the visit. If any imaging or biopsies have been performed, arrangements are made to expedite the delivery of the images, slides, and reports to my office.

During this initial conversation, the patient is also referred to my financial coordinator, Victoria. She will review the patient's insurance information and, based on the patient's expressed reason for coming to see me, will provide a range of possible financial outcomes and expectations, so that there are no surprises at the time of the visit. My staff are so good at performing these functions that it is extremely rare that a patient will cancel an appointment before ever having seen me. You can see and use examples of useful pre-visit materials on our website, FireStarterPublishing.com/ExcellenceWithAnEdge.

Pre-Visit

Three business days prior to the patient's appointment, I will review the schedule with my medical assistant and my financial coordinator to ensure that patients are correctly scheduled into appropriately templated slots. As a result, on my office day, we are all clear about what needs to be done for each patient on the schedule. I will review with Sarah the information that has been obtained and that which is pending. This will also, as you have heard, generate a phone call to the referring physician. If more information is required, my medical assistant will have ample opportunity between now and the appointment to procure it.

Visit

Sarah, the medical assistant, has prepared for the visit, ensuring that all the materials that she has obtained (and I have already seen) are readily available for the time of the visit. In the days of paper charts, the charts were collated, prepared, and stacked in the appropriate order prior to the visit. In our office, we have a completely electronic medical record, so this step is no longer necessary.

The medical assistant and the financial coordinator have already individually reviewed the schedule with the front desk registrar, Freddy, who is prepared in advance for each patient. Freddy knows which patients have balances that need to be collected prior to the visit, which patients have co-pays, and which patients will need to meet with the financial coordinator, Victoria, either before or after the visit. And, of course, the patients have all received this information in advance through a consultation with Victoria by phone.

The front desk registrar has a specific checklist of tasks that have been completed in advance of the office day, including, but not limited to, ensuring that the reception area is tidy, that there are current issues of major magazines in the appropriate place in the magazine rack, that the reception area television is turned on to a cable news channel and is at an appropriate volume, and that our Internet-connected computer is on and available for the enjoyment of our patients and their families.

Freddy also ensures that our electronic picture frame (which has a rotating set of photos and messages outlining the names and experience of all of the staff members with whom the patients will come in contact) is up and running.

A quick aside about this last point: I encourage you to facilitate frequent opportunities for your patients to learn the names of every member of your staff. Some practices give out cards that read, "The front desk registrar's name is Tonya Powers. The financial coordinator's name is Ethan Stone. The medical assistants' names are Alex Miner and Tina Carruthers." Other practices have pre-printed cards with the names of their staff. They can be business cards or something more elaborate.

This accomplishes a number of things.

First, it gives patients comfort and alleviates their anxiety in dealing with people they don't know. Secondly, it gives the staff a sense of ownership or having "skin in the game." And last, and perhaps most importantly, it makes it easier for patients and families to identify staff by name for providing specific positive feedback about them to you, the physician. Then you can actively harvest these compliments ("Has anyone been helpful to you today in the office?") to feed back as reward and recognition. Remember—rewarded behaviors get repeated.

When Mrs. Miller arrives for her visit, she is greeted by Freddy, the front desk registrar. He is not on the telephone or in an exam room, because we have separated responsibility for those functions in order to allow the front desk registrar to focus solely on the patients and their family members in the reception area. Freddy greets Mrs. Miller immediately and warmly to welcome both her and her family to the practice. Freddy tells the patient how long he expects that she will be in the reception area before being brought in to see the doctor.

He has this information readily available because he is in constant communication with the medical assistant. If the patient is waiting in the reception area for more than fifteen minutes, Freddy will go out to the patient and update her and her family regarding the expected duration of the wait from that point forward. He does this using key words he has been specifically trained to use, which are proven to reduce anxiety and increase patient satisfaction.

If yet another fifteen minutes passes, he will again apologize and update the patient. Additionally, he will call our patient advocate who will perform further service recovery. She will give the patient a five-dollar Starbucks or Dunkin Donuts card, offer a sincere apology, and again update the patient about the reason for and expected duration of the delay. She will also follow up with a letter of apology signed by her, the staff, and the physician.

But, of course, none of this happened in the case of the hypothetical Mrs. Miller.

The staff sees me go into the reception area and greet the patient and her family. They observe me using the same behaviors that I ask of them, including the use of AIDET. I manage up the staff, both as a whole and individually by name, with the patient and her family. As a rule, they see me model all of the behaviors that I am asking and expecting of them.

At the end of the visit, I review with the medical assistant and the financial coordinator the specifics of the visit and any follow-up plans. I communicate both verbally and in written form with them what the next steps will be. Both the financial coordinator and the medical assistant have a specific set of steps that they will follow based on what I communicate.

In the case of Mrs. Miller, who will need an ileocolic resection, the medical assistant will review with her all of the logistics leading up to her appearance in the operating room. Mrs. Miller will leave with a stack of information and no additional questions. Similarly, the financial coordinator will review all of the patient's expectations and obligations, both verbally and very clearly in writing. All throughout the process, they will manage up each other and me.

During our regularly scheduled work rounds, in each of the next four to six weeks, Mrs. Miller's name, status, and plan of action will be brought up and reviewed individually with my medical assistant and with my financial coordinator. The goal is to follow this patient's care and her A/R status from office visit to surgery to post-operative follow-up. Almost always this process will continue weekly until, when we bring up Mrs. Miller, the response is, "Done and done." In other words, her care is complete. She has been operated upon and has had her post-operative follow-up. Her billing and collection have been completed.

Pre-Op

In the days leading up to the surgery, the financial coordinator, Victoria, will obtain all necessary authorizations for the hospitalization and the surgery, and will communicate that specifically with the medical assistant, with me, and with the patient. The medical assistant, Sarah, will have numerous interactions with the patient and with the referring physician's office. She will make sure that the referring physician and his staff all know the details and the date of the upcoming surgery. Additionally, Sarah will ensure the communication of all test results in all directions to be sure that each physician's office is up-to-date with the most current information. And she will communicate frequently with the patient to let her know that this has been done.

Two days before the surgery, Sarah will leave a printout of the entire patient packet for my review. She has already checked and ensured that it is complete, but I will serve as an additional check and balance. The entire packet has already been forwarded to the operating room staff and should be available to them as they create their patient chart. Despite this, I will take the entire packet with me, on the day of the surgery, to ensure that there is no delay.

The medical assistant will call Mrs. Miller on the day before the surgery in order to review the final details of the logistics for the following day. Sarah will ask Mrs. Miller if she has any additional questions and will offer to have me call the patient if she requires any answers or even merely reassurance. She wishes her good luck with the surgery and reassures her that she is in great hands.

Peri-Op

On the day of the surgery, Sarah will send me an email with all of the names and numbers of the physicians with whom Mrs. Miller would like me to communicate. This allows me to easily make these calls immediately upon exiting the operating room.

Because Sarah has established such a relationship with the patient, she is, of course, anxious to learn how the surgery went. And of course, in providing this information, I remind Sarah what a great job she did and how important she is to the care of Mrs. Miller and her family, and I thank her for her excellent work.

On a daily basis, I provide my staff with a list of current inpatients and a list of all patients who have been discharged in the previous 24 hours. In this way, we all know who is in the hospital at any given time and how everyone is doing.

Follow-Up

Upon receipt of Mrs. Miller's name on the daily discharge list, Sarah will email me the patient's preferred telephone number so that I can make my post-discharge phone call within 24 to 48 hours. Sarah will often call the patient, as well, in order to see how she is and to facilitate the first post-operative visit.

At the time of the first post-operative visit, Sarah will create a packet for the patient, which includes the operative report and the pathology report for the patient's own records. She does this at the outset of the visit, so that if the patient is waiting for a few minutes to see me, she will have an opportunity to review those documents and ask me questions regarding them. And, of course, Freddy, the registrar, will know in advance whether Mrs. Miller will need to meet with the financial coordinator during the course of this visit.

From beginning to end of this patient interaction, all of my staff are continually reminded of how important a part of the patient care team they are. Although my name is on the surgery, their imprint is equally visible.

CHAPTER 11
THE PATIENT EXPERIENCE
· · · · · · · · · · ·

When Mrs. Miller receives the news that she requires surgery for her Crohn's disease, she is understandably quite upset and anxious. Dr. Stevens gives her my name and phone number and reassures her that I am a specialist in this field, that I have done many, many of these operations, and that I am going to take great care of her. This goes a long way to alleviate her anxiety because she trusts Dr. Stevens. This recommendation is the single most important factor in her decision to use me as her surgeon.

Even so, when Mrs. Miller goes home, she begins to do her research. This does two things for her. First, it gives her something to do. She is still nervous, and will be, until the surgery is finished. Second, this empowers her. She feels that she can control, to some degree, her situation by learning more about it. She is taking the "E" in AIDET into her own hands.

The first thing she does is talk to her friends and family. She asks if any of them have ever heard of me or if they know anybody who has had surgery for Crohn's disease. She also asks them about their experiences at Mount Sinai to be sure that the hospital itself is a great place (which it is).

The next thing she does is sit down at her computer and Google me. When she does this, the first thing that comes up, at the top of the page, is a link to my profile on HealthGrades.com. HealthGrades is a private website created for patients to rate their doctors on a variety of different categories. There is no regulation. There is no oversight. There is simply the ability for any person to rate any physician on these categories. When she clicks on the link, she sees that (at least at the time of this writing) I have a five-star rating. That is the highest possible rating on this site.

On the next page of my profile, Mrs. Miller can find out how patients have rated me on eight individual categories, all of which are related to service, rather than quality of care. In each one of these, I still rate five stars.

She is encouraged by what she reads there, and her anxiety is certainly relieved to some degree. Would the same be true for you? I hope that you periodically check your own HealthGrades profile.

The second thing she is likely to read on Google is a link to an interview that I did recently with the New York Daily News. In the blurb under the link, it describes me as the vice chairman of surgery, someone with 22 years of experience, and an expert in caring for patients with Crohn's and colitis. Whether she clicks on the article or not, there is a positive message.

The third link on her Google search of my name is the link to my profile at the Mount Sinai website. Here, there is a picture of me, background information, and information about my office. She will also see a link to an announcement that Studer Group has conferred its Leadership in Medicine Award upon me. The first page of her Google search is rounded out by links to several articles that I have written in the medical literature.

Contact

When Mrs. Miller calls my office, fully expecting a phone tree runaround, what she gets instead is Sarah's cheerful voice saying, "Good morning, Surgical Associates. This is Sarah. How may I help you?"

Already she begins to relax. She explains that she is a patient of Dr. Stevens and that she needs to make an appointment to see me to discuss possible surgery for her Crohn's disease. And what she hears in reply is something along the lines of, "Don't worry. We're going to take great care of you. Dr. Harris and

Dr. Stevens work together all the time. I've been Dr. Harris's medical assistant for over four years, and I know that you're going to love him."

Once Sarah has learned the nature of the call, she will offer Mrs. Miller a variety of different times in the next two to ten days at which she can be seen. If there is any hint of urgency or the patient asks to be seen sooner, Sarah promises to see what she can do and get back to her a little bit later in the same day. Almost always we will be able to accommodate such a request.

Mrs. Miller will answer a series of questions regarding demographics and insurance information, being reminded periodically about the reason that this information is required. She will be told that we want to make sure that we have accurate information so that we can make her visit as productive as possible, and so that we can help her obtain the quickest and most efficient reimbursement from her insurance company. She will also be asked if there are any other doctors who might have information that would be helpful for this visit.

She is given a whole host of information about the practice, its location, and ways in which she can get here. She is asked about her preferred method of communication, her preferred phone number, and how she prefers to be addressed (e.g., "Mrs. Miller" or "Jane"). If she has email, Sarah will immediately send a packet of information by email for Mrs. Miller to peruse as well as some forms that will need to be filled out, including the intake form on which she can complete her medical history.

Right from the outset, Sarah has informed Mrs. Miller that I am not a member of her insurance panel. Although this is of concern, Sarah immediately assures her that she will have an opportunity to speak with Victoria, our financial counselor, who is excellent at minimizing her cost and with whom she can speak immediately after we have finished getting her information. If the patient wishes, Sarah will transfer the patient to the financial counselor immediately.

Almost always, however, the combination of the initial referral, the patient's research, and the incredibly pleasant interaction that the patient is having with Sarah will allow the patient to get past her initial anxiety and move forward. At the end of the conversation, Sarah thanks the patient and tells her that she is looking forward to meeting her at the appointed time.

Mrs. Miller is then transferred to Victoria, our financial counselor. Victoria greets her warmly and reassures her quickly about the purpose of the conversation. She explains that her role on our team is to ensure that Mrs. Miller's out-of-pocket cost will be as little as possible. That said, she is also very clear about what the expectations are from the patient's individual insurance company and what the patient is likely to have to pay out-of-pocket at the time of the first visit.

Victoria tells the patient that she has been with me for many years, and that she has worked with the patient's insurance company many times. Then she reassures the patient that when she comes to see me, she will have ample opportunity to meet with Victoria again once we decide upon a course of action for her Crohn's disease. And again, Victoria thanks Mrs. Miller for calling and coming to see us, and tells her that she looks forward to meeting her.

Mrs. Miller might also get a call from me. I will often call a patient prior to her initial visit if any of my staff indicate to me that the patient had some specific questions or even sounded particularly anxious about the upcoming visit. During this call, I am able to reassure the patient of my great working relationship with Dr. Stevens, to answer any burning questions, and to reassure her that at the time of our visit, I will guarantee that she and her family will not leave my office with any unanswered questions. The response to such a call is overwhelming. Patients are blown away when such a pre-visit call is made directly by the doctor.

Pre-Visit Phone Call

Two days prior to her scheduled visit, Mrs. Miller receives a call from our automated scheduling system. She hears a scripted message reminding her of her appointment. She is prompted to enter or speak a response, allowing her to confirm the appointment, or to have Sarah call and reschedule. Studies repeatedly show that pre-visit phone calls significantly reduce no-shows and therefore improve operational efficiency. Even if Mrs. Miller confirms the appointment, she is likely to get a call from Sarah on the day before, just to reconfirm. On the day of the visit, if the schedule is running behind, Sarah will call the patient to let her know, so that she can make adjustments to her own plans.

Registration

Mrs. Miller arrives 15 minutes prior to her scheduled appointment time, as per our pre-visit instructions. She is greeted warmly by Freddy, the front desk registrar, who introduces himself by name and lets her know how long it will be before she sees me. Of course, in this case, I am running exactly on schedule. Freddy generally makes Mrs. Miller feel as if she were expected and that we are happy to see her. Instead of just handing her a clipboard, a piece of paper, and a pen, Freddy explains why each of the forms are needed.

Because she has pre-registered and given us all of her information, most of what she reviews has been pre-printed, which further demonstrates that we are on the ball and that we were prepared for her. Mrs. Miller is asked to review all of this information to ensure that it is, indeed, accurate, and that none of it has changed since her phone call with Sarah. Freddy gives her standard release forms and HIPAA compliance statements, explains what they are for and why she's getting them, and asks her to sign the appropriate documents. And when she does, he thanks her warmly once again.

Many practices have their front desk person serve as their primary telephone answerer. It is better to try to separate these functions, allowing the front desk registrar to focus on caring for patients and their families as they arrive in the practice.

When Mrs. Miller is sitting in the reception area waiting to be seen, Freddy asks her if she is comfortable or if she needs anything. She is shown the computer that is there for her use and the magazines that she might read. She might encounter Tiffany, our patient advocate, even if there is not a problem. Tiffany cruises our reception areas and will often round on patients in the manner pre-scribed by Studer Group (e.g., "Were you informed about any delays?" "Did the registration staff introduce themselves to you?" "Is there anyone you would like to recognize?" "Do you have any suggestions that would improve your experience?").

The Visit

A tall, smiling, staggeringly good-looking, well-dressed gentleman in a white coat comes out to greet Mrs. Miller in the reception area. (I warned you this was an idealized encounter.) I introduce myself to Mrs. Miller and to her hus-band and their daughter, who came with her for the visit. I shake hands with each of them and escort them back to my consultation room.

I tell them who I am, that I have been at Mount Sinai for 22 years, and that I specialize in caring for patients with Crohn's and colitis. I tell them that I have reviewed her records and spoken with Dr. Stevens, and already know quite a bit about her. I also say that I am going to ask her a series of questions about what's going on with her Crohn's disease and her general health, because I want to be thorough, and I don't want to miss anything. This takes only a few seconds (no more time than it takes to walk to the back), but has an enormous impact.

Once in the consultation room, I review the intake form that Mrs. Miller has filled out. We first concentrate on the Crohn's disease symptoms she has been experiencing. Then I perform a quick but thorough review of systems, based on a checklist that I have in front of me, which can be scanned directly into her chart. (My intake form contains the necessary documentation for a complete review of systems that satisfies the requirements for billing purposes. Review an example at FireStarterPublishing.com/ExcellenceWithAnEdge.)

I sit across from the Millers, look directly at them, and lean forward in my chair as they are speaking. My phone does not ring. I do not glance at my computer or my watch. My body language tells them that I am here only for them and their benefit.

Next, I invite Mr. Miller and his daughter to remain in the consultation room while I go with Mrs. Miller to the exam room. At this point, Sarah magically appears to accompany us into the room. This is the first time that they have met in person, so I introduce them and manage up Sarah. (More often than not, patients are so excited about meeting Sarah for the first time that they are managing her up to me.)

Everything in my actions and my interaction with Sarah demonstrates to Mrs. Miller that I consider Sarah to be an extremely valuable part of our team who is caring for her, rather than as a servant or an inferior.

In the exam room, I make sure to cover Mrs. Miller, and to tell her that I am doing so for her privacy. I wash my hands, and I tell her that I am washing my hands so that they are clean when I examine her. These are both examples of "key words at key times" to connect the dots for her about why I am doing what I do, so she understands the purpose of my actions. My explanations also reinforce these behaviors in her mind, alleviating any anxiety that she might have about her privacy and about cleanliness in my office. Furthermore, these words and actions serve as a trigger for her, if and when she fills out a patient satisfaction survey in the future.

Again, as I examine her, I tell her what I am doing, why I am doing it, and what my findings are. There is nothing worse than silence in aggravating the anxiety of an already nervous patient.

I return to the consultation room with Mrs. Miller and again greet her family. This time, I review the findings to-date, and, using drawings and analogies often tailored to the patient's own profession, review all of the options available. I do not limit myself to all of the reasonable options, but instead review the universe of options available in this situation. Those that are clearly untenable, we dismiss together immediately. (This exercise is worthwhile, so that the patient and her family understand that you have thought about all the possibilities prior to making any kind of decision.)

Often (if not usually), there are two equally legitimate options remaining on the table. We spend a lot of time reviewing all of the risks and the benefits of each of these two options, making sure to allow the patient to interject with comments or questions along the way. This does not slow you down. Quite the opposite. It ensures that the patient understands the options and their implications, and is able to articulate them back to you. All questions are answered, and together we agree upon a plan, pending, of course, the approval of Dr. Stevens. I reiterate, at this time, that Dr. Stevens remains a critical part of the decision-making team and of her care.

When all of the questions have been answered and the plan has been established, I escort the Millers back to the reception area, shake all of their hands, and thank them for coming (the "T" in AIDET). I also encourage them to call again if there are any further questions that they have. I seat them in the reception area and let them know that both Sarah and Victoria, the financial counselor, will see them shortly to review any logistics and any financial issues that are expected to arise. This is an opportunity for me to greet the next patient and his or her family. Invariably, there is no one else in the waiting room besides the Millers and the next patient I am scheduled to see.

Checkout

At this point, Mrs. Miller is satisfied that there is a plan that she fully understands, and that all of her questions have been answered. There are, however, the logistics to be worked out. I have made it very clear to her that Sarah and Victoria will help her manage the logistics and the finances.

First, Sarah brings the Millers to a private area in order to discuss the logistics of the coming surgery. She reviews with them a whole host of information that she will also give to them in printed form. For examples of some of these, see the website, FireStarterPublishing.com/ExcellenceWithAnEdge.

This information not only includes details such as the preparation for the surgery, but also includes post-operative information such as a list of foods that are encouraged and/or are prohibited, so that the Millers can do the appropriate shopping before she enters the hospital for her surgery. Sarah again reassures them that they are in great hands and manages up Mount Sinai and me at every opportunity.

Next, Victoria, who has been given the specific codes for the operation that Mrs. Miller will undergo, reviews the financial details with the patient and her family. This includes the specific CPT codes that will need to be conveyed to the insurance company. Additionally, having performed this surgery many times in the past, we have a sense of history with Mrs. Miller's insurance company, and we can guide her as to what the typical reimbursement is and what her out-of-pocket costs are likely to be.

At this point, many practices will ask for a certain percentage of the professional fee to be paid prior to a procedure. There are certainly pros and cons to this approach. After resisting this for many years, I have found that there is great value to my practice in collecting at least a portion of my fee prior to surgery. (In fact, I am quite happy to write a refund check to a patient when the combination of her preoperative payment and the insurance payment exceeds my fee. It means we have been very effective at billing and collecting.)

Two or three days after the visit, Mrs. Miller is likely to receive a phone call from me. I tell her that I am calling to follow up and to make sure that she has no further questions or concerns since I saw her. Clearly, in the hour we spent together, I imparted a tremendous amount of information to her, and much of it may have been overwhelming to her.

My experience is that a patient is extremely grateful for this call and that only one or two questions arise. I also have found that patients who have seen multiple physicians and obtained multiple opinions will commit during this call to using me as their specialist. However, it is important to remember that the purpose of this call is to provide excellent care. It is not a sales call. Patients can always discern the difference.

Pre-Operative Preparation

Mrs. Miller will receive a number of communications from my office. Sarah will continue to ensure that all of the information required for the surgery has been obtained and will continue to inform Mrs. Miller about the status of our information.

Additionally, Victoria, the financial coordinator, will keep Mrs. Miller and her family informed about the status of the authorizations required for the upcoming surgery. If at any point the patient expresses a desire to speak with me, or if any questions arise that my staff cannot answer, this will generate a phone call from me to the patient.

On the day before the surgery, Sarah will again call the patient to confirm the specific time that she is expected in the hospital, and to go over any last-minute questions and/or information that is required. During these days prior to the surgery, Sarah really is Mrs. Miller's best friend.

Day of Surgery

I have reassured the patient and her family that on the morning of surgery I would see her well before the operation. Mrs. Miller sees me as soon as she arrives in the pre-operative holding area. At that time, I ask her if she has any additional questions. I address each member of her family, and reassure all of them that she is in experienced hands, that I will take care of her as if she were my own family, and that the second that I am finished with the surgery, I will personally come and see the family members and let them know that she is finished, that she is well, and that the surgery has gone as planned.

All are reassured by this interaction. I personally introduce Mrs. Miller to my anesthesiologist and reassure her that we have worked together many, many times. A note of caution here: Due to the nature of our system, and the inability to control all variables, there are times when either the nursing team or the anesthesiologist with whom you are working is not one with whom you are completely familiar. This is true not only in surgery, but in a variety of team situations throughout tertiary care medicine.

Because of this, I caution you against introductions in front of a pre-operative or pre-procedure patient. All interaction, both verbal and non-verbal, must indicate to the patient that this is a finely honed, experienced team that has worked together numerous times and operates as a well-oiled machine.

Anything less is extremely anxiety-provoking. Don't say things that are not completely true, but you should not draw attention to the fact that you don't often work together. Over the years, I have a number of times corrected an anesthesiologist, a medical student, or a nurse for introducing him or herself to me in front of an awake, pre-operative patient.

Keep in mind that one of the fruits of practicing excellence with an edge is enhanced control over your working environment, maximizing the likelihood that you will be working with your own team most of the time.

I remain with the patient until she is asleep, all the while managing up the hospital and the personnel who surround her. Although Mrs. Miller is unaware at the time, the moment the surgery is finished and I have reviewed the results with her referring physician(s), I go personally to the family waiting room to discuss the outcome with the patient's family. Of course, I have obtained permission to do so prior to the surgery. While I see many physicians call the waiting area by telephone, I think this is a huge mistake.

I go downstairs and individually greet each of the patient's family members. I review the specifics of the operation and reassure them that their loved one is doing well and that the surgery was successful. Of course, if there were any untoward events, I review them immediately in a non-defensive and non-threatening manner.

Later that day, Mrs. Miller will receive a visit from me, usually while in the recovery room. Of course, given the amnestic effects of the medication she has received, she may not remember this visit. This does not diminish its importance.

Hospital Stay

Mrs. Miller will receive numerous visits each day of her hospital stay. She will be seen by my house staff at least twice, by me (or my partner) at least once if not twice, and rounded on hourly by the nursing staff. Each one of these visits is an opportunity to alleviate anxiety and to manage up each of the other members of the team caring for her. Any occasion to round together with the house staff, the referring physician, and/or the nurses is to be celebrated.

During each one of these visits, I will sit down, whether it is in a chair, on a window ledge, or on the patient's bed. And I will end every visit with the opportunity for Mrs. Miller to ask me any questions that have not been answered to-date. She will invariably thank me, to which I will respond either, "My pleasure," and/or, "Thank you for allowing me to care for you."

Discharge Day

On the day that Mrs. Miller is scheduled to be discharged from the hospital, I will again sit down and review her instructions. I am very specific with regard to activity, showering and bathing, proper hygiene, diet, wound care, driving, and expectations for post-operative visits. I consistently use the same language every time to ensure that I do not miss anything.

Additionally, Mrs. Miller will receive written instructions including a specific list of dietary instructions. I will review all of her prescriptions with her, and at that point reassure her that I have been speaking with Dr. Stevens and that he is on board with our plan. On that day, of course, I will call him.

Within 48 hours, Mrs. Miller will receive a call from me. I have done this for the entirety of my career with every single patient every single time. I have found that my patients are extremely grateful that I call and that it reconfirms that they are not merely names on my list. These calls give me an opportunity to clarify any instructions and to answer any other questions that they might have. Again, many studies have shown that these post-visit phone calls improve patient compliance, increase patient satisfaction, and enhance loyalty. They also significantly reduce the number of phone calls that come into the practice from post-operative patients.

Post-Operative Visit

When Mrs. Miller comes for her first post-operative visit, she is given an envelope that contains the dictated operative report and her pathology report. She is instructed that these are for her own records. She is reassured that all of her doctors have already received copies of the same. She is given an opportunity to read and review these while she is waiting. It gives her an opportunity to formulate questions prior to seeing me.

When I see Mrs. Miller, I offer to review any questions that she might have with regard to these reports. I again reassure her that her physicians all have copies of the reports, and that I have reviewed her course with them. And I use this opportunity to manage up the referring physician(s) and reassure Mrs. Miller that she is in great hands for her ongoing care.

At the end of this visit, I express my pleasure at the outcome and my thanks for her trust in me to care for her and her family. And I assure her that, although I do not need to see her again for my own benefit, I am always available for either a phone call or a follow-up visit if any further issues or questions arise. I also tell her that all of our interactions will be imparted to her referring physician so that his records are complete.

At this visit, Mrs. Miller will also see Victoria, who has already called her in advance to review the status of her financial account. Victoria will update the patient about any correspondence or receipts from the insurance company, and will gently remind Mrs. Miller of her obligations. None of this is a surprise to the patient. Victoria reassures Mrs. Miller that we will continue to work with her and the insurance company in order to ensure that we can quickly conclude the financial part of our interaction and minimize her out-of-pocket costs.

When she leaves the practice, Mrs. Miller is not only grateful and satisfied with the care that we have provided, but equally as important, she is extremely pleased with her own physician for having facilitated our intervention. She will certainly go back to Dr. Stevens and thank him for what he has done. She is at this time even more loyal to him, and as a result, he is more loyal to me as a consultant for his patients.

LIVING EXCELLENCE WITH AN EDGE

· · · · · · · · · ·

In the end, *living* excellence with an edge is about being a better doctor. If you are Affable, Able, and Available and show your patients, your staff, and your referring physicians the care and respect with which you would treat your own family and friends, the rest will take care of itself. You'll enjoy healthy market share, positive financials, and the benefits of a skilled and talented staff.

I never said it was easy, though. Reaching daily for excellence can be hard work, but it *is* doable. It is also rewarding and is teachable to others. Any physician can use the tools I have just shared to replicate my success and get similar results. He or she will hardwire excellence with an edge in any practice.

Over the years, I have found that doing the right thing for patients is invariably the right thing for my staff, my referrers, and my bottom line. Perhaps the greatest compliment I have ever received was from a graduating chief resident giving a speech to a roomful of his teachers, mentors, and juniors. He said, "Whenever I am in a difficult situation—whether it's in the operating room, talking to a patient, or sharing news with a family—I ask myself, *How would Mickey handle this?*"

My advice, of course, is: "Be a mensch!" Put the patient first, and you, too, will achieve success. You will be the whale in your waters. And, more importantly, you will continually be reminded of the impact you have on the lives of your patients and their families, as you receive letters like this one…

Dear Dr. Harris,

It's been two weeks and a day since you operated on Connie. To say thank you just wouldn't have been enough, so I wanted to try to express not just for me, but for my family, just how we feel.

Over the last two years, watching Connie suffer with Crohn's disease hasn't been easy. Her slow deterioration was very difficult to watch. Everyday life was a battle. Over the last two weeks, I have watched her come through the surgery, and her recovery has been a difficult, yet joyful, experience.

When Connie decided to have this operation, she had consulted with Dr. Itzkowitz to recommend a surgeon. You were top on his list. From her first meeting with you, she <u>knew</u> you were her surgeon. You made Connie and our family so comfortable with an understanding of the procedures and what to expect with the outcome. Your comforting yet honest approach during this most difficult time was, needless to say, very reassuring.

After surgery, we had a conversation at the nurses' station. Your excitement for Connie's prognosis was a moment I'll always remember, for you understood what this surgery meant to her quality of life. Your excitement was that bedside manner, that human quality, humor, and professionalism.

Now, two days before Christmas, we have already had our gift. Dr. Harris, your team of doctors and all the people you work with have been absolutely the best. I wish you all that you ever want, and all that you ever need in life. To you, your family, friends, and staff: May God bless you all.

Sincerely,
Farley, Connie, Matthew, and Kevin Kemler

BIBLIOGRAPHY

· · · · · · · · · ·

1. Source: SK&A, A Cegedim Company, Irvine CA April 2010.

2. Grote, Kurt D., John R. S. Newman, and Saumya S. Sutaria. "A Better Hospital Experience." *McKinsey Quarterly*. November 2007. (19 July 2010).

3. Johnson, Avery, Jonathan Rockoff, and Anna Wilde Mathews. "Americans Cut Back on Visits to Doctor." *The Wall Street Journal*, 29 July 2010, sec. A.

4. "Capturing Lost Revenues." *Health Care Advisory Board Cost and Operations Presentation 2002*. The Advisory Board, 2002.

5. Chang, J.T., et al. "Patients' Global Ratings of Their Health Care are not Associated with the Technical Quality of their Care." *Annals of Internal Medicine,* 144, no. 9 (2006): 665-72.

6. Bauer, M., et al. "Hospital Discharge Planning for Frail Older People and Their Family. Are We Delivering Best Practice? A Review of the Evidence." *Journal of Clinical Nursing* 18, no. 18 (2009): 2539-46.

Dudas, V., et al. "The Impact of Follow-Up Telephone Calls to Patients After Hospitalization." *Dis Mon* 48, no. 4 (2002): 239-48.

7. Forster, A. J., et al. "The Incidence and Severity of Adverse Events Affecting Patients after Discharge from the Hospital." *Annals of Internal Medicine* 138, no. 3. (2003): 161-67.

8. Phillips, A., C. Vincent, and M. Young. "Why Do People Sue Doctors? A Study of Patients and Relatives Taking Legal Action." *Lancet* 343 (1994): 1609-13.

9. Goyal, Deepi G., et al. "To sit or not to sit?" *Annals of Emergency Medicine* 51 (2008): 188-93.

10. Beale, E., et al. "Impact of physician sitting versus standing during inpatient oncology consultations: patients' preference and perception of compassion and duration. A randomized controlled trial." *Journal of Pain Symptom Management* 29, no.5 (2005): 489-97.

11. Kane, Carol K. "The Practice Arrangements of Patient Care Physicians, 2007-2008: An Analysis by Age Cohort and Gender." *Policy Research Perspectives, American Medical Association*, 2009.

12. Center for Patient and Professional Advocacy at Vanderbilt and Studer Group. *Unprofessional Behaviors in Healthcare*. 2009.

13. Stoller, Gary. "Companies give front-line employees more power". *USA Today*. 26 June 26 2010. (19 July 2010).

14. Griffin, Jill. Customer *Loyalty: How to Earn It, How to Keep It*. San Francisco: Jossey-Bass, 2002.

RESOURCES

· · · · · · · · · · ·

Accelerate the momentum of your Healthcare Flywheel˙.
Access additional resources at FireStarterPublishing.com/ExcellenceWith-
AnEdge.

STUDER GROUP COACHING:

Studer Group˙ coaches hospitals and healthcare systems providing detailed
framework and practical how-tos that create change. Studer Group coaches
work side-by-side establishing, accelerating, and hardwiring the necessary
changes to create a culture of excellence. In our work, Studer Group has iden-
tified a core of three critical elements that must be in place for great organizational performance once a commitment is made to the pillar approach to goal
setting and the Nine Principles˙ of Behavior.

Emergency Department Coaching Line
Is a comprehensive approach to improving service and operational efficiency
in the Emergency Department. Our team of ED coach experts will partner
with you to implement best practices, proven tools, and tactics using our
Evidence-Based Leadership^{SM} approach to improve results in all five pillars—
People, Service, Quality, Finance, and Growth. Key deliverables include
decreasing staff turnover, improving employee, physician, and patient satisfaction, decreasing door-to-doctor times, reducing left without being seen
rates, increasing upfront cash collections, and increasing patient volumes and
revenue.

To learn more about Studer Group coaching, visit StuderGroup.com.

BOOKS: categorized by audience

Senior Leaders & Physicians

Leadership and Medicine—A book that makes sense of the complex challenges of healthcare and offers a wealth of practical advice to future generations, written by Floyd D. Loop, MD, former chief executive of the Cleveland Clinic (1989-2004).

Engaging Physicians: A Manual to Physician Partnership—A tactical and passionate roadmap for physician collaboration to generate organizational high performance, written by Stephen C. Beeson, MD.

Straight A Leadership: Alignment, Action, Accountability—A guide that will help you identify gaps in Alignment, Action, and Accountability, create a plan to fill them, and become a more resourceful, agile, high-performing organization, written by Quint Studer.

Physicians

Practicing Excellence: A Physician's Manual to Exceptional Health Care—This book, written by Stephen C. Beeson, MD, is a brilliant guide to implementing physician leadership and behaviors that will create a high-performance workplace.

All Leaders

The HCAHPS Handbook: Hardwire Your Hospital for Pay-for-Performance Success—Three Studer Group experts—Quint Studer, Brian Robinson, and Karen Cook, RN—explore the significance of HCAHPS to our industry's future and offer specific tactics aimed at helping hospitals achieve and sustain improved results on each survey composite.

Hardwiring Excellence—*A BusinessWeek* bestseller, this book is a road map to creating and sustaining a "Culture of Service and Operational Excellence" that drives bottom-line results, written by Quint Studer.

Results That Last—*A Wall Street Journal* bestseller by Quint Studer that teaches leaders in every industry how to apply his tactics and strategies to their own organizations to build a corporate culture that consistently reaches and exceeds its goals.

Hardwiring Flow: Systems and Processes for Seamless Patient Care—Drs. Thom Mayer and Kirk Jensen delve into one of the most critical issues facing healthcare leaders today: patient flow.

Eat That Cookie!: Make Workplace Positivity Pay Off...For Individuals, Teams, and Organizations—Written by Liz Jazwiec, RN, this book is funny, inspiring, relatable, and is packed with realistic, down-to-earth tactics to infuse positivity into your culture.

"I'm Sorry to Hear That..." Real Life Responses to Patients' 101 Most Common Complaints About Health Care—When you respond to a patient's complaint, you are responding to the patient's sense of helplessness and anxiety. The service recovery scripts offered in this book can help you recover a patient's confidence in you and your organization. Authored by Susan Keane Baker and Leslie Bank.

What's Right in Health Care: 365 Stories of Purpose, Worthwhile Work, and Making a Difference—A collaborative effort of stories from healthcare professionals across the nation. This 742-page book shares a story a day submitted by your friends and colleagues. It is a daily reminder about why we answered this calling and why we stay with it—to serve a purpose, to do worthwhile work, and to make a difference.

<u>101 Answers to Questions Leaders Ask</u>—By Quint Studer and Studer Group coaches, offers practical, prescriptive solutions to some of the many questions he's received from healthcare leaders around the country.

Nurse Leaders and Nurses

<u>The Nurse Leader Handbook: The Art and Science of Nurse Leadership</u>—By Studer Group senior nursing and physician leaders from across the country, is filled with knowledge that provides nurse leaders with a solid foundation for success. It also serves as a reference they can revisit again and again when they have questions or need a quick refresher course in a particular area of the job.

<u>Inspired Nurse</u> and <u>Inspired Journal</u>—By Rich Bluni, RN, helps maintain and recapture the inspiration nurses felt at the start of their journey with action-oriented "spiritual stretches" and stories that illuminate those sacred moments we all experience.

Emergency Department Team

<u>Excellence in the Emergency Department</u>—A book by Stephanie Baker, RN, CEN, MBA, is filled with proven, easy-to-implement, step-by-step instructions that will help you move your Emergency Department forward.

For more information about books and other resources, visit FireStarterPublishing.com.

MAGAZINES:

<u>Hardwired Results - Issue 11, 2009</u>
Tools to create accountability and add dollars to your bottom line

Hardwired Results - Issue 12, 2009
Offers a wealth of evidence-backed insights on addressing the three "As"—
Alignment, Action, Accountability—to achieve peak performance.

Visit StuderGroup.com to view additional *Hardwired Results* magazines.

ARTICLES:

Keep Your Patients Coming Back
MGMA Connexion
August 2008

Quint Studer on 5 Important Issues Facing Healthcare Leaders
The Hospital Review
November 14, 2008

Unlocking the FEAR Foothold
Quint Studer
March 2009

Evidence-Based Leadership
Projects@Work
Quint Studer

How to Achieve and Sustain Excellence
Healthcare Financial Management

To read these articles and view other resources, please visit StuderGroup.com.

SOFTWARE SOLUTIONS:

Leader Evaluation Manager™: Results Through Focus and Accountability
Studer Group's Leader Evaluation Manager is a web-based application that automates the goal setting and performance review process for all leaders, while ensuring that the performance metrics of individual leaders are aligned with the overall goals of the organization. By using Leader Evaluation Manager, both leaders and their supervisors will clearly understand from the beginning of the year what goals need to be accomplished to achieve a successful annual review, can plan quarterly tasks with completion targets under each goal, and view monthly report cards to manage progress.

To learn more, please visit FireStarterPublishing.com.

INSTITUTES:

Taking You and Your Organization to the Next Level with Quint Studer
Learn the tools, tactics, and strategies that are needed to Take You and Your Organization to the Next Level at this two-day institute with Quint Studer and Studer Group's Coach Experts. You will walk away with your passion ignited, and with Evidence-Based Leadership℠ strategies to create a sustainable culture of excellence.

Nuts and Bolts of Operational Excellence in the Emergency Department
Improve patient flow and build service and operational excellence in your Emergency Department as Jay Kaplan, MD, FACEP, and Stephanie Baker, RN, CEN, MBA, both with extensive and ongoing real-life ED experience, share proven tactics such as Provider in Triage, Rounding for Outcomes, Discharge Phone Calls, Key Words at Key Times, and AIDET℠.

Resources

• • •

What's Right in Health Care^{SM}
One of the largest healthcare peer-to-peer learning conferences in the nation, What's Right in Health Care brings organizations together to share ideas that have been proven to make healthcare better.

To review a listing of Studer Group institutes or to register for an institute, visit StuderGroup.com/Institutes.

For information on Continuing Education Credits, visit StuderGroup.com/CMECredits.

Visit FireStarterPublishing.com/ExcellenceWithAnEdge to access and download many of the resources, examples, and tools mentioned in *Excellence with an Edge*.

ACKNOWLEDGMENTS
· · · · · · · · · ·

I have really enjoyed the process of writing this, my first book. If you like it, it is because of the people listed below and many, many others. If you do not, it's all me.

There are three groups of people I would like to acknowledge—those who inspired *Excellence with an Edge*, those who made it possible, and those who made it happen.

In the first group, of course, are all of the patients and their families who have honored me by entrusting me with their care. So, too, are all of the doctors who have referred these patients to me. I have tried to make you glad that you made such referrals. Working with me as a part of my team are all of the non-physician professionals and staff, who come to work every day with the same motivations as I do—to practice excellence with an edge. I have also been inspired by all of my partners, past and present, with special thanks to the late Irwin Gelernt (the big guy), to Steve Gorfine (the mensch), and to Sergey Khaitov (my not-at-all-junior young partner). I have to thank all of my teachers and mentors, of which there are too many to list, but I need to single out the one who inspired me to become a surgeon in the first place, my chairman, Michael Marin.

Quint Studer really made this book possible, along with BG Porter and the rest of the Studer Group® team. The idea came about in an animated discussion with Quint, when I told him that in a competitive environment like New

York, you have to have an edge. Here, I said, you have to practice excellence *with an edge* in order to thrive. Quint's response was, "That's the title of your book. Now go write it!"

"Go write it" required a lot of help. Deb Wallis converted my midnight ramblings into the printed word. My editor, Chris Roman, turned that printed word into coherent prose. Sara Harris (no relation) somehow turned my napkin scribbles into lovely graphics. And Debbie Harris (yes, relation) helped soften the edges to make the book more readable and to keep me out of trouble. The stories she removed will almost certainly appear in the book we'll write *after* I retire. Finally, Bekki Kennedy and her team from Fire Starter Publishing and Dottie DeHart and her staff at DeHart & Company put the whole thing together in such a way as to make me say, "Wow, it actually looks like a real book!"

I thank you all.

ABOUT THE AUTHOR

. . . .

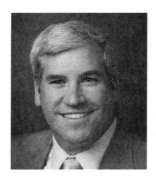 Michael T. Harris, MD, is a nationally recognized expert in the field of gastrointestinal surgery, particularly in advanced reconstructive surgical techniques for inflammatory bowel disease (Crohn's disease and ulcerative colitis). He has helped pioneer the use of minimally invasive (laparoscopic) surgical techniques for both diseases and has one of the largest IBD practices in the nation.

Mickey (only his mother calls him "Dr. Harris") received his undergraduate degree from Cornell University in 1984, studying Russian literature. He went on to earn his medical degree from the College of Physicians and Surgeons at Columbia University in 1988. He completed his general surgery residency at Mount Sinai and then was managing partner of a large private surgical practice for over 10 years. Mickey was awarded the Association of Attending Staff/Bella Trachtenberg Award in 1993 as Mount Sinai's most outstanding chief resident across all services.

Dr. Harris has been very active in support of The Mount Sinai Medical Center. He is currently an officer of the Hospital Medical Board and its Executive Committee, and serves on the Board of Governors of Faculty Practice Associates, the 840-physician multispecialty group of The Mount Sinai School of Medicine. As the elected president of the Association of Attending Staff, comprised of over 2,000 active clinicians at Mount Sinai, Mickey served as a strong advocate for patients and their physicians. He is currently on the Steering Committee and is the lead physician champion for Mount Sinai's Studer Initiative. His own practice has consistently scored in the 99th percentile nationally on the Press-Ganey patient satisfaction surveys.

In 2007, Mickey was awarded with the Mount Sinai Department of Nursing's highest honor for physicians, the Physician of the Year Special Recognition Award, given for outstanding collaboration with Mount Sinai nurses.

Dr. Harris was recently made a vice chairman of the Department of Surgery at Mount Sinai, responsible for the management of Surgical Associates, a 45-surgeon faculty practice. He was recruited to this position and charged with helping create the premier patient-centered multispecialty surgical group in the nation.

At The Mount Sinai School of Medicine, Dr. Harris created and is the course director of the popular "Business of Medicine" elective, one of the first courses of its kind for medical students in the country.

In 2009, Dr. Harris was awarded the National Leadership in Medicine Award by Studer Group' and a Gold DOC Award from the Arnold P. Gold Foundation for humanism in medicine.

How to Order Additional Copies of

Excellence with an Edge:
Practicing Medicine in a Competitive Environment

Orders may be placed:

Online at:
www.firestarterpublishing.com
www.studergroup.com

By phone at: 866-354-3473

By mail at: Fire Starter Publishing
913 Gulf Breeze Parkway, Suite 6
Gulf Breeze, FL 32561

(Bulk discounts are available.)

Excellence with an Edge
is also available online at www.amazon.com.